NURSE MANAGER ENGAGEMENT

STRATEGIES FOR EXCELLENCE AND COMMITMENT

BARBARA L. MACKOFF, EdD

Visiting Professor of Nursing
Adelphi University
School of Nursing
Garden City, New York

JONES AND BARTLETT PUBLISHERS
Sudbury, Massachusetts
BOSTON   TORONTO   LONDON   SINGAPORE

World Headquarters

Jones and Bartlett Publishers
40 Tall Pine Drive
Sudbury, MA 01776
978-443-5000
info@jbpub.com
www.jbpub.com

Jones and Bartlett Publishers
Canada
6339 Ormindale Way
Mississauga, Ontario L5V 1J2
Canada

Jones and Bartlett Publishers
International
Barb House, Barb Mews
London W6 7PA
United Kingdom

Jones and Bartlett's books and products are available through most bookstores and online booksellers. To contact Jones and Bartlett Publishers directly, call 800-832-0034, fax 978-443-8000, or visit our website, www.jbpub.com.

Production Credits

Publisher: Kevin Sullivan
Acquisitions Editor: Amy Sibley
Associate Editor: Patricia Donnelly
Editorial Assistant: Rachel Shuster
Production Editor: Amanda Clerkin
Marketing Manager: Rebecca Wasley
V.P., Manufacturing and Inventory Control:
    Therese Connell

Composition: Shawn Girsberger
Cover Design: Scott Moden
Cover Image: © Palto/ShutterStock, Inc.
Printing and Binding: Malloy, Inc.
Cover Printing: Malloy, Inc.

Library of Congress Cataloging-in-Publication Data

Mackoff, Barbara.
  Nurse manager engagement: strategies for excellence and committment / Barbara L. Mackoff.
      p. ; cm.
  Includes bibliographical references and index.
  ISBN-13: 978-0-7637-8533-8
  ISBN-10: 0-7637-8533-4
  1. Nurse administrators. 2. Leadership. I. Title.
  [DNLM: 1. Nurse Administrators. 2. Leadership. 3. Models, Nursing. 4. Nurse's Role. 5. Nurse-Patient Relations. 6. Physician-Nurse Relations. WY 105 M1665 2011]
  RT89.M29 2011
  362.17'3068—dc22
                            2010003934
6048

Printed in the United States of America
15 14 13 12 11   10 9 8 7 6 5 4 3 2

Dedicated with love and honor to Selma Sadie Mackoff

ॐ ॐ ॐ

A magnificent mother and nurse manager

Contents

Acknowledgments

This book belongs to the exceptional nurse managers on these pages. They have revealed the habits of heart and mind to teach us the art of engagement.

I can't imagine the Nurse Manager Engagement Project (NMEP) taking wing without Dr. Pamela Klaus Triolo, my clinical partner, who was there from the first draft of the budget, the online IRB testing, the strategic selection of study sites, the marathon analysis sessions, word searches, and the final proofs of the study's journal submissions. Pamela—I am so grateful for your seasoned perspectives, generous insight, and oversight.

Special thanks to Sue Hasmiller, Senior Project Manager at the Robert Wood Johnson Foundation (RWJF), for her initiation of the NMEP, and to our project manager Michelle Larkin, who navigated the project through RWJF. My appreciation to Adam Coyne for connecting all of the dots, and to Barb Farrell and M. T. Meadows at the American Organization of Nurse Executives (AONE) for the opportunity to teach, and learn from, so many nurse managers.

It was a pleasure to work with AONE as a publishing partner. I especially want to acknowledge Pam Thompson, AONE Chief Executive Officer, for her support and generativity, and Kim Cavaliero, AONE Senior Communications Specialist, for her savvy stewardship of the book's completion. Special thanks to Emily Ekle at Jones and Bartlett Publishers for her vision and verve, and to Rachel Shuster and Amanda Clerkin for keeping me on target.

And thank you, Jeremy and Hannah, my best beloved cheerleaders.

About the Author

Barbara Mackoff, EdD, is a consulting psychologist, author, and leadership educator with a strong focus on the demands of nursing practice. She is a visiting professor at the Adelphi University School of Nursing in New York, and a core faculty member of the Nurse Manager Fellowship Program of the American Organization of Nurse Executives.

Dr. Mackoff was the principal investigator of a national research study of nurse manager engagement funded by the Robert Wood Johnson Foundation. She is on the faculty of the University of Colorado's Rocky Mountain Leadership Program and has been a scholar-in-residence at both Massachusetts General Hospital and Brigham and Women's Hospital in Boston. Her bold approach to leadership is in demand by healthcare organizations across the country, including the American Organization of Nurse Executives, the Nursing Leadership Academy, the National Association of Healthcare Executives, Baylor Healthcare, US Healthcare, Providence Hospital, University of Washington Hospital, AtlantiCare, Portland Children's Hospital, Jackson Hospital, Baltimore Franklin Square Hospital, Houston Methodist Hospital, and the M. D. Anderson Cancer Center.

Dr. Mackoff's research has been published in the *Journal of Nursing Administration* and *Nurse Leader* magazine. She is the author of five highly praised books that have been published in five languages, including *The Art of Self-Renewal.* She is also co-author of *The Inner Work of Leaders: Leadership as a Habit of Mind.*

Dr. Mackoff graduated cum laude from Tufts University, received a master of arts degree in teaching from the University of Massachusetts, and master and doctoral degrees from Harvard University. She has held educational and clinical appointments at Tufts University, Northeastern University, and the University of Washington Medical School and Department of Psychiatry and Behavioral Sciences.

Dr. Mackoff's perspectives on leadership and productivity have been described in her appearances on *The Today Show, CBS Morning News, CNN,* and *All Things Considered.* Her work has also been profiled in the *New York Times, USA Today,* and the *Washington Post.*

Foreword

Since 1967, the American Organization of Nurse Executives (AONE) has provided leadership, professional development, advocacy and research to advance nursing practice and patient care. Through these efforts, AONE has played an active role in promoting nursing leadership excellence and shaping health care public policy. Our goal is to equip nurse leaders with the latest research, tools and resources available to assist them in their professional development.

Dr. Barbara Mackoff has spent many years working with nurse managers through classes, seminars, research projects and interviews—gathering information about why nurse managers do the important work that they do. Dr. Mackoff continues to research the many factors that compel nurse managers to work in this rewarding, yet difficult field.

This book is based on research conducted by Dr. Mackoff in a national *Nurse Engagement Study*. Rather than focusing on issues of attrition, dissatisfaction and data from exit interviews—as has been the focus of many research studies in the past—Dr. Mackoff's groundbreaking research places the focus on why nurse managers stay in their jobs. This book offers an exciting new look at an old problem by focusing on methods to keep nurse managers engaged, energized and enthusiastic in their roles and incorporating these positive steps into nursing education, professional development and recruitment.

The nurse leaders interviewed for this book provide an enlightening look at the nursing workforce today. Their stories are honest and thought provoking. I hope you enjoy reading this book and will take away new knowledge and inspiration to help you in your career as a nurse leader.

Pamela A. Thompson, MS, RN, CENP, FAAN
AONE Chief Executive Officer

CHAPTER 1

Begin in the Middle

This book began four summers ago in a spirited conversation about nurse middle managers with Sue Hassmiller, a senior program officer at the Robert Wood Johnson Foundation. Sue asked, "How do we keep middle managers from leaving?" I responded, "One way to answer that question might be to talk to the nurses who stayed—the long-term and outstanding managers—not the ones who left."

"Can you write a grant to study that idea?" Sue wondered. "Yes," I said, and picked up the phone. My call went to my colleague Pamela Klauer Triolo, who was chief nursing officer and associate dean, academic–service partnerships at the University of Pittsburgh Medical Center, who joined me as a clinical partner in this project.

The result was the *Nurse Manager Engagement Project* (NMEP), which was fully funded by the Robert Wood Johnson Foundation (RWJF). This two-year study was conducted at six of the United States' top medical centers and involved interviews with 30 nurse managers—exemplars of both longevity and excellence.

The clear intention behind our focus on middle managers was to address the math of the current urgent and complex nursing shortage. It is one in which the aging boomers meet health care's Bermuda Triangle of staff nurse vacancies, middle manager attrition, and retirement-bound nurse leaders.

The enormity and complexity of this problem can lead to a circular chicken-and-egg trope. (Where do we start?) Guided by Sue Hasmiller's questions and several established research trends, we began in the middle—with nurse managers. The NMEP was grounded in the consideration of three related ideas that underline the critical role of the nurse middle manager:

- Staff nurses' satisfaction is linked to their relationship with their manager.
- Future nursing leadership comes from development of middle managers.
- Nurse manager satisfaction and longevity are currently at an all-time low.

This trio of ideas suggests that it is no longer enough to explore our failures to retain nurse managers in their work. Instead, a fresh paradigm is needed to approach this meaningful middle. Our goal with the NMEP was to design a study that would challenge previous research designs for examining manager vacancies—ones that focused on attrition, dissatisfaction, and data from exit interviews. The mission demanded a change of both the vocabulary and the focal question.

RETENTION VERSUS ENGAGEMENT: A METRIC OR A MODEL?

One icy Boston morning at Massachusetts General Hospital, I had breakfast with a group of medical–surgical nurses. I asked them to set aside their coffee and danish to draw two pictures: one of nurse retention and the other of nurse engagement. Their retention drawings featured symbols of restraint: a ball and chain, a locked gate, a dike holding back water. In contrast, the engagement images depicted connection and emotional content: hands held, eye contact, listening with pleasure.

I gave the same assignment several months later in a San Diego seminar attended by 30 nurse manager fellows from the American Organization of Nurse Executives (AONE). One manager drew retention as a paper clip and engagement as big ears. In another drawing, retention was golden handcuffs festooned with dollar signs and engagement was a golden heart.

One intriguing way to think about these drawings is to recognize that they mirror the root meanings of the words retention and engagement. Retention is derived from the Latin verb *retinere*, which means to hold back, keep, or restrain. By contrast, the roots of engagement lie in the French verb *engager*, defined as holding the attention of, to give one's word, to honor or commit.

The drawings also portray the static nature of retention and the dynamic nature of engagement. They underline David Cooperrider's (1995) suggestion that "words create worlds." A fresh approach demands a careful choice of words. Previous studies of nurse manager retention have been grounded in deficit-based problem descriptions. These reports of dissatisfaction and attrition are becoming as familiar as the nursing shortage statistics. As the exodus of nurse managers becomes an increasingly urgent aspect of the current nursing shortage, it is imperative to use vocabulary that implies solutions rather than problems.

The idea here is not to retire the word retention, but rather to recycle it and to reduce its footprint by using it as a metric rather than a model. This requires a focus on building an exemplary and solution-based model of both longevity and excellence for nurse managers.

An exemplary model can be captured in the word engagement. As a beloved business buzzword, this term has attracted researchers who have conducted several large-scale studies on the topic, including those by Gallup (2006) and Harter and Schmidt (2007). In these studies, employee engagement is characterized as a deepened emotional connection that an employee feels for the organization—one that influences the employee to work with superior productivity and job performance.

The research also links engagement and retention, with 85% of engaged employees indicating that they planned to stay with their employer through the next year. This linkage suggests that any effective nurse retention strategy must be built on an understanding of engagement. The creation of an exemplary model of nurse manager engagement, as compared to a metric attrition/retention count, would have powerful implications for nursing graduate education, job descriptions and recruitment, organizational self-study/development, and continuing nursing education.

The notion of engagement in the NMEP was defined in terms of exceptional work and longevity. This study gathered data from in-depth interviews with 30 nurse managers in six hospital settings. Each participant was nominated by senior leadership based on two criteria: five or more years as nurse manager and designation as outstanding in her or his work.

ENGAGEMENT AS POSITIVE DEVIANCE: WHY DO SOME NURSE MANAGERS STAY?

A shift in approach to study engagement rather than retention also demands a change in the focal question. Instead of asking why nurse managers were leaving, our study identified 30 high-performing nurse managers at six outstanding medical centers with five or more years' tenure and asked them why and how they were engaged in their practice. The research posed two related questions: (1) Why do nurse managers stay? and (2) What are the individual and organizational elements that are associated with successful long-term tenure of nurse middle managers?

This approach is consistent with what Jerry Sternin (2003) calls "positive deviance." Sternin, founder of the Positive Deviance Institute at Tufts University, believes that solutions are always present in the problem situation. He has grounded his applied research within one actionable premise: *In every orga-nization of people with the same function, there are certain individuals who function more effectively—and who have resolved the problem.* Innovative problem solving takes place when communities discover the successful uncom-mon behaviors of these positive deviants.

There are three pillars of positive deviance that support the creation of a model of nurse manager engagement:

- The solutions are present in the situation.
- In every community, there are positive deviants—people who have resolved the problem.
- You can't clone people but you can capture their wisdom and adopt their successful strategies to create an exemplary model.

By applying this approach, the study of outstanding long-tenured nurse managers—positive deviants in a field where nurse manager attrition was the norm—ensured that its results could be used to build an evidence base of engagement. Such evidence can, in turn, be used to create an exemplary model that describes behaviors of engaged individuals and the culture of engagement in their organizations. From this model, applications can be designed to allow others to practice these behaviors.

In addition to the positive deviance model, the NMEP had two other anchor-ing inspirations. First, the study drew upon the work Gratton and Ghosol (2005), who had used the term *signature behaviors* to describe the factors that embody the positive values, characteristics, aspirations, and interests of individuals and their organizations. Second, the appreciative inquiry methodology as described by David Cooperrider (1990) was applied to create a self-report instrument, the *Nurse Manager Engagement Questionnaire* (NMEQ), to elicit signature ele-ments linked to engagement.

The appreciative inquiry approach—like Sternin's positive deviance model—is a solution-centered methodology that is grounded in the idea of seeking out the positive behaviors of individuals and organizations. As Cooperrider explains, "It is a search for the best in people, their organizations, and the relevant world around them. In its broadest focus, it involves systematic discovery of what gives 'life' to a living system when it is most alive, most effective, and most con-structively capable."

For Cooperrider, the questions we ask are fateful because they drive the solutions we find. As a practical matter, this means that the question, "What is wrong?" must be replaced by the question, "What is working?" This effort may include the following elements:

- Crafting of the unconditional positive questions that lead to solutions rather than negation, criticism, and diagnosis
- Asking people to talk about past and present capacities—achievements, assets, unexplored potentials, innovations, strengths, elevated thoughts, opportunities, benchmarks, high point moments, lived values, traditions, strategic competencies, stories, expressions of wisdom, insights into the deeper corporate spirit or soul, and visions of valued and possible futures

The NMEQ tool was used to harvest data on signature individual and organizational elements that revealed reasons outstanding managers stayed in their role. The interview questions, which were designed to be asked as part of one-on-one interviews, focused on unconditionally positive questions to discover the experiences, strengths, and enduring values of engaged individuals and organizations. Among the key topics were the following:

- Beginnings: initiation into the role
- Self-reported strengths
- Positive factors that influenced the decision to stay
- Satisfactions and high point experiences
- Organizational role in success and longevity
- Aspirations: wishes and perceptions of a positive future for the nurse

The NMEQ interview questions were tested in a pilot group interview with five long-standing nurse managers at the University of Texas Medical Center in February 2006. The questions were then shaped into final form to be used in the six healthcare settings covered by the study (**Figure 1–1**).

Through a synthesis of positive deviance and appreciative inquiry methodology, the NMEP study involved four steps:

1. **Define** what successful solution would look like. The study defined engagement as longevity (five years or more as a nurse manager) and excellence (as designated by the participant's selection by the chief nursing officer).
2. **Determine** whether any individuals already exhibit this behavior. Chief nursing officers in six organizations were asked to nominate five nurse managers with five or more years of experience in the role who exhibited excellence in their management role.
3. **Discover** uncommon practices. The NMEQ's positive questions were employed to discover signature elements of individuals and organizations that contribute to engagement.

4. **Design** interventions that allow others to practice these new behaviors. The findings were used to suggest applications in evaluation and education and organizational development.

---

1. Let's talk about your beginnings as a middle manager at _____ medical center. What were your first positive impressions or promising or satisfying experiences in the first few weeks or months?
2. What did you learn during that early time that has helped you succeed over the years in the role?
3. You have been in your role at _____ for at least five years. How do you explain the positive factors that have influenced your decision to stay in your job?
4. What gifts, values, attitudes, and capabilities do you bring to the challenges of being a nurse middle manager? How have these allowed you to be successful, and to work long term, in this role?
5. What do you bring to the middle manager role that allows you to connect with so many different people—patients, families, nurses, and administrators?
6. What is satisfying and gratifying about your experience of middle management in this setting? What do you contribute day-to-day that gives you a feeling of pride?
7. Describe a stand-out or high point experience in this setting—a time when you felt most engaged and alive. What made it such a memorable experience? Who was involved? What part did you play?
8. Your collaborative relationship with staff nurses contributes to high-quality patient care. Describe a time when your partnership with a nurse made a difference in the care of a patient. Which factors were present? What did you contribute?
9. Your interface with administrators and senior leadership is essential to your own leadership. Give an example of a time when an administrator or senior manager helped you succeed. What was happening? Who was involved? What was the outcome?
10. How has this particular organization been a good fit in enhancing your success and longevity as a middle manager?
11. Recall a time when you felt supported by your organization. What happened? Who was involved? Which conditions were present?
12. If you could be granted three wishes for new middle managers coming into the field, what would you wish for them?
13. Imagine this: As you drive home from work today, you slip through a wrinkle in time. It is the year _____. All of the vacancies for nurse managers across the country are filled, the average tenure of a nurse manager is 10 years, and nurse manager satisfaction is among the highest in the nursing field. What has happened to create this change?

Figure 1–1   Nurse Manager Engagement Questionnaire (NMEQ)

THE DATA OF ENGAGEMENT

The study participants comprised 30 nurse managers in six hospital settings (**Table 1–1**). Each participant had been in a management role for more than five years and was designated as outstanding in her work (**Table 1–2**). In addition, the nurse leader who selected the participants in each setting filled out a questionnaire about their choice of the nurse manager. The dominant themes in their selection are summarized in Chapter 4.

During the spring and summer of 2007, I conducted 29 interviews at the six participating medical centers and one interview by telephone. Using the NMEQ tool developed for the study, each of the 1½-hour audio-taped interviews consisted of open-ended, guided questions, weighted toward the appreciative

---

Table 1–1   Locations of Nurse Manager Engagement Study

- Cedars-Sinai Medical Center (Los Angeles, California)
- Children's Memorial Hospital (Chicago, Illinois)
- University of Pittsburgh Medical Center/Shadyside (Pittsburgh, Pennsylvania)
- Seton Medical Center (Austin, Texas)
- NYU Langone Medical Center (New York, New York)
- University of Washington Medical Center (Seattle, Washington)

Table 1–2   Description of Participants in Nurse Manager Engagement Study

Age	Years in Nursing	Years at Facility	Years in Position	Highest Degree Earned
35–40 (8)	5–10 (1)	5–10 (7)	0–5 (5)	AD (1)
41–45 (2)	11–15 (4)	11–15 (4)	6–10 (14)	BSN (12)
46–50 (10)	16–20 (7)	16–20 (6)	11–15 (5)	Master's (17)
51–55 (6)	21–25 (6)	21–25 (6)	16–20 (6)	PhD (0)
56–60 (4)	26–30 (8)	26–30 (6)		
	31–35 (4)	31+ (1)		

Notes: $N = 30$ female nurse middle managers. The numbers in parentheses are the numbers of participants in each group.

inquiry approach. The participants received the questions in advance. The inter-view questions were designed to elicit high point experiences, enduring values, and signature positive behaviors in individuals and organizations that contribute to engagement of nurse managers.

Working together, my clinical partner Pamela Triolo and I analyzed 45 hours of taped interviews and 600 pages of transcripts. Narrative analysis was used to harvest signature individual and organizational elements associated with nurse manager engagement as well as larger ideas across the various dimensions. The data analysis procedure included the following steps:

1. All interview tapes were transcribed.
2. A list of major individual signature themes was identified from each indi-vidual transcript.
3. Lists of dominant themes in each organization were assessed from the five individual interviews from that organization.
4. A list of dominant themes across all six organizations were noted and ranked in order of occurrence.

Significant themes and subthemes were noted across all protocols. The analysis shaped a model of nurse manager engagement as a busy intersection between individual signature elements and elements of culture and organization.

INDIVIDUAL SIGNATURES

Ten signature elements were clear dominant themes in the interviews with the 30 outstanding nurse managers. These behaviors, capabilities, and attributes of long-term individual nurses managers are summarized in **Figure 1–2** and are described in detail in Chapters 2 and 3.

The analysis divided the ten elements into two categories: those linked to *line of sight* (LOS; the ability to link management role with nursing mission) and those linked to *emotional mastery* (EM) of the unique challenges of the nurse manager role:

- Mission driven (LOS)
- Generativity (LOS)
- Ardor (LOS)
- Identification (LOS)
- Boundary clarity (EM)
- Reflection (EM)
- Self-regulation (EM)
- Attunement (EM)
- Change agility (EM)
- Affirmative framework (EM)

Signature Element Characteristics	
1. **Mission driven (LOS)** "It's the patient; it's the person in the bed."	• Directs orientation toward purpose and intention • Focuses on end result and outcome while addressing day-to-day operational concerns • Defines context with big-picture thinking to frame and explore specific issues
2. **Generativity (LOS)** "I love seeing my birds fly."	• Finds gratification and joy in development of others • Creates a legacy in the nurse manager's own image • Maintains continuity and linking generations • Offers and grants opportunities for autonomy and freedom
3. **Ardor (LOS)** "I cannot begin to explain to you how energized I am every morning—because I will be working with this group."	• Conveys excitement about staff, colleagues, and leadership • States dedication to patient care • Declares commitment to the organization
4. **Identification (LOS)** "Everything that I take pride from comes from how the floor runs."	• Describes and savors the nurse manager's part in the accomplishments and success of the nursing staff • Maintains a clear line of sight that connects the nurse manager's own work to the care of the patient at the bedside • Creates an atmosphere where staff can provide superb patient care
5. **Boundary Clarity (EM)** "If I took it as a personal attack, I would never survive."	• Cultivates strong internal boundaries • Creates emotional insulation • Restores boundaries through disengagement • Models and displays appropriate boundaries

Figure 1–2 Ten elements of individual engagement

6. **Reflection (EM)** "It's the self-awareness and being careful that I don't lose people working with me."	• Leverages lessons from experience • Observes the effect of the nurse manager's behavior on others • Scans for cues about self and others in workplace
7. **Self-regulation (EM)** "Sometimes it's learning when *not* to say something."	• Uses restraint to keep emotions in check • Practices perseverance • Cultivates patience • Suspends judgment before acting
8. **Attunement (EM)** "I am always going to get their side of the story—before jumping to conclusions."	• Shows regard for the individual and appreciation of each person's contribution to the organization • Understands diverse perspectives and standing in another person's shoes • Sets aside assumptions to hear the whole story
9. **Change Agility (EM)** "I am usually the first to try something."	• Challenges the process through innovation • Welcomes and initiates change • Seeks change through new learning
10. **Affirmative Framework (EM)** "If you stay with the negativity and complaining, the staff will see that your hair is on fire."	• Uses an optimistic explanatory style • Generates positive expectations • Models resilient behavior

LOS = line of sight; EM = emotional mastery.

Figure 1–2   Ten elements of individual engagement *(continued)*

Although the signature elements of emotional mastery and line of sight reso-
nate throughout the data, they are expressed in ways as individual as handwrit-
ten signatures. Contrast the two narratives of Tuyen K., a nurse manager in a
large community hospital, and Susan R., a manager in a metropolitan children's
medical center.

When Tuyen K. arrived in the United States from Vietnam 34 years ago, she
enrolled in college two weeks later. She taught herself English with the words
in her math textbook. This experience became a template for her *emotional
mastery* of change. As she explained:

> Yes, in a situation that you're put in, you can do it. I always go back and think
> what will make me confident or brave. To do what I have done reflects back to the
> time when we left our country and came here. That was a huge impact in my life
> because if you could overcome that you can do anything.
>
> I look back and ask myself, "How did you do it?" That's why I say, there is no
> doubt about my attitude. Ever since I've become a nurse, ever since I've been in
> this country, because you have nothing but to look forward to do things. . . . The
> people I work with, not many people when they give me a task ask me if I can do
> it. . . . I would take it and say, "Give me some direction." That's what I learned, I
> guess, just from the way I was brought up in my family and our culture and expe-
> riences I've been through. You take it, you do it, you're still not sure, you go back
> and ask questions, and then you move on with that.

In her interview, Tuyen also revealed her *line of sight*—her capacity to be
an effective manager and stay connected with the mission of nursing care at
the bedside:

> I bring my best to work. Every day—and this is what inspires me—I have tried to
> mentor other people on my staff. Every day, I look at me and say, "Whose life are
> you going to make better or easier today?" And if I can fulfill that, it doesn't matter
> if it's big or small, it really doesn't matter; it's the best that I can do for that day.

Susan R., a former flight nurse and director of paramedics in Chicago, was
introduced to nursing by working as a ward clerk in a "big crazy emergency
room" while she was in school to become a teacher. "I never thought nursing
would be for me," she recalled.

> When people would walk into the emergency room and they were full of blood, I would
> have to go throw up, every single time. The nurses would say, "Don't go in there."
> . . . The physicians were the ones who said I needed to get over this and pretty
> much took me by the hand. The next step in the ER was to be an aide. I went
> through the course and then I moved on to be a tech. By the time I became a tech,
> I thought I would like to be a nurse, too. I managed to finish two degrees in seven

years from two different schools. I absolutely loved it. I took other courses in emergency medicine to see if I could actually do this and loved it.

When Susan described her setting (a children's medical center), she revealed her *line of sight* to patient care: "The kids are the best. That is so fun to be a part of. I love coming here. I live far away and I'm never sad that I have to come to work." She elaborated:

I'll tell you the kids come first, and it begins with each of us. We have service principles that we share with the staff. Some of it is basic—being polite—and some of it is extending yourself; some of it is putting yourself in the shoes of these families, or the children, or your employees, so that you can work with them to achieve their goals. It's very important to me to be able to teach other people and to help them grow. I don't mind if people leave me to go on to do bigger and better things—I love it actually. I feel like I've done my job and they have grown and they make me proud. I keep in touch with them. That's my philosophy.

One observation I made when I first got here was I expected to walk in the emergency room and hear crying kids constantly—and you won't. You might hear one or two, but you will not hear more than that. Usually we make more noise than that talking amongst ourselves. That is why I know that we go the extra mile to make sure the children are comfortable. I've never seen the extension for children here in any other job. If we have to haul a child with his IVs down the hall into the room where the refrigerator is so he can pick out his own popsicle, we will do it because that's one of the few choices children get and they want to do it themselves.

Susan also explained how lessons from her varied experiences allowed her to be a successful change agent—with the *emotional mastery* to understand multiple perspectives:

[I have] been a ward clerk, an aide, and a tech in the emergency department, and a student nurse in an ICU. I have worked as a nurse in the ER and on a flight program, which I oversee here, the transport teams, being the director for the paramedics for the city of Chicago, working in collaboration with the city of Chicago politics, three resource hospitals and their politics. All these things have prepared me very well to do what I do now. It's not black and white; it's really always gray. There are always different perspectives that play in a lot of decision making that, had I not done these things, I would think that things are still black and white—and they're not. I think that opens me up to be successful here because I get that. My staff sometimes doesn't get it. They'll ask, "Why can't we just do it this way?" I show them the issues that play into the decision and give them some background on how you actually get a process done. This helps me the next time something changes. I'm very good at explaining changes because I've lived it.

SIGNATURES OF ENGAGED ORGANIZATIONS

Five signature elements of organizations that contribute to excellence and long-term commitment of nurse managers were consistently mentioned during the 30 interviews (**Figure 1–3**). Notably, four of these five signature cultural elements were aligned with individual signature elements.

- Learning culture
- Culture of regard
- Generative culture
- Culture of meaning
- Culture of excellence

These elements are described in-depth in Chapter 5. Although each health-care environment was unique, the five signatures of cultures of engagement were echoed from coast to coast. Listen to Tuyen and Susan describing the cultures of their organizations.

Susan explained her attraction to her organization as a *culture of regard* that communicates her value and the value of nursing expertise:

So at the center of all that is that it's a good fit, because in this organization, people realize how much you bring to it, and they listen and they turn to you and respond to suggestions that you make, knowing that they are coming out of this whole backlog of experience . . . I feel that they have invested in me. I think they believe that I am a good thing for their ER, and they've invested in me. So I have had great opportunities to do things that I never in my wildest dreams knew I would be doing. They had me participate in some focus groups for [posters in] emergency rooms—never done that prior to coming here. I didn't think the things I did were worthy of those, when in fact they were really quite cool.

Susan also details specific examples of how her organization conveys esteem through responsiveness to her viewpoint and decisions:

I used to be a flight nurse for a helicopter, and I've been the director of the para-medics for the city . . . when I came here, I was very concerned about the safety issues we were having or could have with that ambulance and heli-pad. I was taken extremely seriously about that, and they let me implement [my suggestions] because I could explain to them what needed to be fixed and why. They let me be the negotiator for the contracts. I felt like, "You should tap into this background

Learning Culture "The greatest learning and growth opportunities have been being able to participate in projects or initiatives that are beyond the unit's goal and to really be involved in something bigger."	• Creates opportunities for educational mobility • Encourages learning through risk taking and increased visibility • Provides transparency of information and resources
Culture of Regard "He turned to me and the medical directors and said, 'You know how to run your department; you know what you need.' He handed me, verbally, a virtual blank check for 13 more full-time employees."	• Conveys esteem for nursing through responsiveness to the viewpoints and decision making of nurse managers • Fosters collegial physician–nurse relationships and accountability • Empowers nursing practice; facilitates goal attainment
Culture of Meaning "In everything that I have tried to do or have done, the question is always, 'Is it the best thing for children and their families?' No matter who is in the president's role, if they ask that question, there is some sense that they believe it, too."	• Fosters alignment of individuals' and the organization's goals and values • Communicates with clarity about the organization's mission and values
Culture of Generativity "Her goal was to make sure that everybody was competent enough to work without her, and that is my goal. If I'm in a car accident tomorrow, they need to survive, the patients need to do well. For me, if I don't do that, I am sending them out to fail."	• Encourages the use of visible mentors or designated preceptors • Provides exemplars to serve as role models • Offers available and approachable senior leadership
Culture of Excellence "We joke about it, but 98% is never good enough."	• Cultivates brand pride in the organization's accomplishments and reputation • Communicates high standards and expectation of excellence

Figure 1–3   Signatures of engaged organizations

I have, because I really am knowledgeable; I could cite you the EMS act, and this would work to our advantage"—and they totally let me. I felt like the stuff I came with, we got to use it. Disaster planning, emergency medicine, prehospital stuff, transport—they definitely turn to me for advice. Gordon, the [chief operating officer], will call me at home with questions, and I like that, and I like to be able to utilize that.

Tuyen offered an unforgettable scenario of her organization as a *culture of meaning*, with an emphasis on the recognition of religious values of the patient and the willingness to meet each patient's needs:

We have brought a monk to perform the ritual prayers. I was moved by that. We have patients who are dying, and I worked with them and with the sisters [nuns]. It was, "What do you need? We need to support you." They [would] run around and get all the stuff that people needed. I have started to remember; I always want to cry when I remember.

We had one family [who] just came in here and asked if I could help to translate. When the father expired in ICU, they did a little prayer, a little ritual. I could feel their resistance. I asked, "When do you want me to call the funeral home? Do you have arrangements?" They never did answer my question. I finally pulled one of the daughters to the side and asked, "What is the next step? What do you want us to do?" She finally said, "We want to perform our ritual, a little bit of gold to put underneath his tongue and a little rice." They believe this [death] is another journey so they need to give him food.

Well, I thought, "Where do we get the gold?" One of the daughters said, "I can go home and scrape it off from one of my rings at home." We got another cab and sent her home. The kitchen was closed, and we needed some rice. I asked someone to go to the kitchen and get some rice. He got two steps away and asked, "How much?" I didn't know, so I said, "Just get a bowl." He got three steps away and asked, "Cooked or uncooked?" Every time, it was another question. I asked the daughter, "Do you want cooked or uncooked?" She said, "Uncooked." So he finally came with a big bowl of rice—he must have picked the biggest bowl in the kitchen. Well, they only took one grain of rice and put in his mouth. The daughter came back and put a little gold in his mouth. So we were able to fulfill their request.

Tuyen captures her organization's culture of meaning when she says, "It's integrity with respect and wisdom. To me, wisdom is the integration of all that. The bottom line is really not the religious practices but the patient's needs. That's how I look at it."

AFTER THE STUDY: BUILDING THE EVIDENCE BASE

In the three years since the formal NMEP study was completed, I have had the opportunity to meet with hundreds of nurse managers around the country and engage them in an ongoing and vital dialogue about the theory and practice of nurse manager engagement. Among them were the managers I met as a visiting scholar at Massachusetts General Hospital in Boston, as a faculty member of the Nurse Manager Fellowship Program of the American Organization of Nurse Executives (AONE), and at a seminar with an AONE-sponsored group of outstanding managers involved in the Robert Wood Johnson Foundation's *Transforming Care at the Bedside* (TCAB) initiative. Several of these meetings created opportunities to gather more data, including data submitted by the 60 AONE nurse manager fellows and 30 TCAB nurse managers who filled out the Nurse Manager Engagement Questionnaire (NMEQ) in written form.

Examples and data from these groups are included in this book with an important caveat: The criteria for the selection of the TCAB group and the AONE nurse manager fellows differed from the criteria used to select the 30 managers in the original study. Each of the two groups met the criteria of excellent performance by virtue of their selections to participate in these programs. However, they did not all meet the "five years on the job" criterion of the NMEP. Although a majority of the TCAB managers were long-time nurses, many AONE fellows—though they were chosen for their excellence—were only a few years into the role.

The chapters that follow will describe the formal findings of the original NMEP study. That said, the rich conversations and written questionnaire data from the TCAB managers and AONE fellows have served to validate and deepen the initial evidence base of the original study in terms of the behaviors of individuals and their organizations linked to nurse manager engagement. For this reason, the additional data are also included in discussions in this book. Examples from the original study will be designated as "from the NMEP"; the later data are noted as "TCAB managers" and "AONE fellows." Other verbal anecdotal examples will be referred to by city of origin.

For those readers who want to chew on the scenery or bring this book to class, the book also includes a glossary and three full interview transcripts.

The portraits and particulars of engaged nurse managers described on these pages are instructive, mirthful, provocative, and moving. By offering vital data about their individual and organizational strengths and aspirations, these exceptional managers provide exemplary models for further research and exciting application. Their observations offer readers a tool of reflection about what it means to be a nurse manager.

CHAPTER 2

Individual Behaviors Linked to Line of Sight

My first lesson about the importance of *line of sight* for nurse managers was at a meeting of the Nursing Advisory Counsel. During the question-and-answer segment, Doris E. told a story about an event that became a commitment. On a day that was aging her in dog years, Doris escaped from her office for a walk. She passed a staff nurse with her knees bent—to establish eye contact with a pediatric patient. She recalled this illuminating moment:

> Watching our nurse I realized: This it is what we really do. At the end of the day, my work contributes to the person at the bedside providing a patient with excellent care. We get so busy keeping the rocks off the road that we get misaligned. It was four years ago, but I can still see that nurse.

I was reminded of Doris in a marathon meeting with my clinical partner Pamela Triolo, as we poured over the data for patterns. One of the earliest themes that emerged was the importance for managers of being able to see the link between management behavior and bedside care. As Pamela observed, "That's where we go wrong. We stick nurse managers in meetings all day and block their line of sight to the patients."

The concept of *line of sight* (LOS) has been used to describe how an individual understands the way his or her day-to-day work contributes to the larger vision, values, and objectives of the organization (Boswell & Boudreau, 2004). In the NMEP study, managers spoke of the loss of the ability to see their impact on direct bedside care of patients as the elephant in the middle of the room for nurse managers.

In the study, the engaged nurse manager's capacity to maintain the LOS between his or her management work, patient care, and organizational mission emerged as a critical—and previously under-documented—aspect of long-term nurse manager engagement. The four signature individual behaviors noted in the NMEP study were *mission primacy, identification, ardor,* and *generativity.* Each signature was linked to maintaining a clear LOS between the nurse manager role and the values that originally attracted these individuals to bedside nursing. The four signatures have also been consistently underlined by hundreds of nurse managers in conversations and classrooms.

MISSION DRIVEN

The focus on the big picture and the organization's overall mission is one of the biggest changes in making the move from the role of staff nurse to the role of manager. As one nurse manager admitted, "The owl in me is very good at the small stuff—the nuts and bolts. But I have to think big. I have to have a vision of where I want to be, what I want to be doing or how I want to change things."

- Directs orientation toward purpose and intention
- Focuses on the end result and outcome while addressing day-to-day operational concerns
- Defines the context with big-picture thinking to frame and explore specific issues

Mission statements, which are designed to create a framework of meaning and shared values, are a foundation in nursing practice environments (Girard, Linton, & Bestner, 2005). In the NMEP study, managers from five of the six hospitals could be characterized as motivated and driven to action by a sense of meaningful mission.

The managers in that study and those I have interviewed and taught express this signature element in several consistent ways.

They Maintain Orientation Toward Purpose

Leadership educator Warren Bennis (1989) described the capacity to be oriented toward purpose as "the management of attention." It is the process that enables nurse managers to remind themselves of why they do what they do.

Summaries of this purpose have been voiced in many settings: "It is the patient; it is the person in the bed." "I am committed to veterans' care." "It is a part of my job to get the staff to remember the purpose of their work."

Examples from Interviews

It's just amazing. It's amazing because even with all the technology, all the medicines, all the procedures, it still comes down to sitting at that bedside, holding someone's hand when they are in their lowest moment, and I see that on a daily basis.

But it's all about the patient. All my decisions are based on the patient, because that is why we are here. Again, that keeps me very focused; that keeps me [in a] "follow the rule" mentality. It's all about the patient, and we have to figure it out if the patient is unhappy and why. Or we have to figure out what we could have done differently in this patient's continuum of care. There is always a choice. It may not always be the choice we want, but there is always a choice.

We didn't have a nurse's aide; it was me who worked with this patient. It was a slow day. I took a basin and soaked her feet and pampered her feet. That was the best thing I could do for that patient that day. You go back to TLC, the "touch"—that's what you really have in nursing. Whatever I do, there is always a purpose. If you do something and you don't have a purpose, you're not going to be successful. It's wonderful when you have a purpose.

They Focus on Outcome

Organizational consultant and poet David Whyte (2001) defines the focus on desired outcome as "the discipline of memory." It is the ability to recall what is most essential while addressing day-to-day operational issues. Managers talked about "focusing on what needs to be done, as well as multitasking" and "learning to think about what I really wanted as a outcome." One manager explained her outcome on focus with a green analogy, saying, "Do the onerous tasks first. You have to weed the garden before it can grow and flourish."

Examples from Interviews

One of the things that I bring is that I am able to figure out what the outcome is that I want. It isn't fame; it isn't fortune; it's not notoriety or even acknowledgment. In many ways, it really is about understanding what is the right thing to do and can I figure out how to get there—and I almost always can figure out the right thing and I can almost always figure out how to get there. [It] doesn't always work completely smoothly. I'm only human, and most of the time I can do that. It really matters to me to do the right thing; it matters to me intensely to do the right thing, and I will do the right thing even when it is seriously unpalatable. There are gross things that you have to do as a manager, like invite people to not be in their positions any longer or things like that, that are really, really icky—and yet it's the right thing and that's my job. So I'm willing to do what is unpleasant when it's right for my responsibilities and for the unit as a whole and for these patients.

> I think it's where we want to be and how can we get there—not focusing on the process (although the process is important), but I would first start with what is it that we are trying to achieve and then how do we get there. Sometimes we actually back it up and go forward. I think that it's assuming that everyone is there to accomplish the same thought and has the shared goal and is there to accomplish it.

They Define Context with Big-Picture Thinking

Nurse leader Carolyn Mills (2005) defined *context* as taking into account how the bigger picture relates to a specific issue, and understanding the limits and opportunities of operating in a complex organization. "I think the longer you are in this role, you see a bigger and bigger picture," suggested one manager.

Examples from Interviews

> I am good at prioritizing, but I think big—that big perspective. I'm always looking for meaning. I look at the data; I'm looking for the meaning in the data. I look at an interaction; I'm looking for the bigger picture of the process again. What's going on here? I always have a vision of where I want to be or what I want to be doing or how I want to change things.

> I think there were times when things weren't going well, maybe where the team wasn't working as well together as I thought it should be. They weren't getting along. There were those times when I wanted to give up, and yet I looked and thought, "No, I can do this, I can get through this." What I remember is that if I stayed focused on the bigger picture and the broader perspective of why I was in the role and why I wanted to continue, that helped me to then not focus on the little petty things, even though they are little and yet significant, but to stay focused on the bigger picture.

GENERATIVITY

A nurse manager, who was fond of metaphors and being a mentor, bought a sponge in the hospital gift shop—the kind that grows to 10 times its original size when wet. "When this gets big enough to take over my job, I'm done.

- Enjoys growth of others
- Creates legacy in own image
- Builds links between generations
- Offers autonomy

I am growing a boss," she said. From coast to coast, managers expressed the gratification in watching the growth and success of their staff.

These engaged nurse managers suggested a signature element that went beyond descriptions of nurse mentoring (Olson, 2002; Wilson, 2005). The word "generativity," as defined by psychologist Erick Erikson (1950, 1982) and expanded by McAdams (McAdams & de St. Aubin, 1992; McAdams, Hart, & Maruna, 1998), can be used to describe the capacity of nurse managers to find pleasure and satisfaction in caring for and contributing to the next generation.

Through the practice of generativity, nurse managers can establish a clear LOS to the care at the bedside. In the NMEP, nurse managers in five of the six organizations described themselves in terms of generativity. Subsequent discussions with other managers also underscored the importance of the four distinct facets of generative behavior that were harvested from the original study.

They Experience and Express Pleasure in the Growth and Development of Others

The capacity to find satisfaction and enjoyment in watching others grow is described by Erikson (1950) as a favorable balance of creativity and productivity over stagnation and self-absorption. Studies of nurse/mentor relationships have noted nurses' inclination toward generativity (Byrne & Keefe, 2002). As one nurse manager exalted, "I just love helping people get where they want to be." Recently, a nurse manager of two decades from Indiana described her pleasure in her staff's growth: "My high point in middle management is when one of my staff expresses joy in an accomplishment or when a new nurse passes his or her boards—knowing that our encouraging and training has helped."

Examples from Interviews

Our nurses are just so bright. They go from being a new grad to running a committee by themselves or going to great lengths to make something different for a patient and figuring stuff out, and we get to recognize people and present them with awards toward things. To see that growth is one of the best parts of the job, to have visible improvements in how the workload goes—just to feel like things are getting better all the time and I can look at the nurse and say, "I'm here to support you; you know that's my role." To have them be able to see things get better. If something happens and one of my RNs is going to get the credit, I just sit back and enjoy that. I just love to see that growth.

I think it's watching other people grow and knowing that you are a part of that. Over the course of my tenure as a manager, we've grown my specific one unit from 14 beds to 22 beds, so there was a time where we had 17 or 20 new graduates all at one time. [I enjoy] being able to be that supportive person not only to the new graduates, but to their preceptors, and watching someone evolve as an educator/preceptor/mentor to the brand-new person, as well as watching those green people grow into a good, solid practice.

They Create a Legacy in Their Own Image
In the NMEP study, descriptions of generativity—depicted as creating a legacy—inspired many avian analogies. Two favorites: "I see myself imprinted on them, almost like a mother duck" and "I love seeing my birds fly." Generativity was also described in terms of teaching, training, and sharing skills with a younger generation. These actions create meaning at work and serve as an extension of self that will outline the nurse manager's own presence on the job (Kotre, 1984; McAdams & de St. Aubin, 1998). A manager from Iowa explained, "I have high expectations and nurture and encourage my staff to grow. I encourage them to do the right thing even though there may be some cost to us."

Examples from Interviews

> I mentor them, so they can one day be me. I think I have the right people on the bus but they have to believe that. It's very important to me to be able to teach other people and to help them grow. I don't mind if people leave me to go on to do bigger and better things; I love it actually. I feel like I've done my job and they have grown and they make me proud. I keep in touch with them. That's my philosophy.

> On a personal level, it gave my ego strokes because it was validating: Yes, I really do know this, and I am helping someone else. I like to help people. I get my kicks from helping people, whether it is helping them succeed or helping them get better. This was just more global. I could reach more people by doing that. I like helping new nurses begin. To this day, that has never dimmed. That is probably the favorite part of my job. I really, really like getting the new ones in here and getting them started and giving them the enthusiasm that I have.

They Maintain Continuity and Link Generations
The responsibility for preparing future generations and passing on the culture/meaning systems of an organization (McAdams, Hart, & Maruna, 1998; Valiant & Milofsky, 1980) was integral to expressions of generativity. Remember the manager who was "growing a boss?" Like many of her peers, she reveals a strong emotional investment in the strategic process of succession planning.

Examples from Interviews

> [It is] believing in the new generation's ability to care for me and my children as we age; to have the knowledge that my time in nursing was worth it. That [when] I do leave, not only from this job, but from so many jobs and so many patients, that I can still remember back to by name, by sight; to know truly in my heart that I have made

a positive difference. I am at the crux now of getting ready in succession planning to leave management and prepare others to want to step into this job. Nurse managers across the country talk about the fact that nobody wants our job.

Nobody is applying for these nurse manager jobs; we are burning ourselves out. The younger people are looking at the number of hours we work and don't want any part of it. . . . I am preparing them. Because I have told them about succession planning and because they see what I'm doing, I have nine assistant nurse managers who, if I was to leave tomorrow, maybe not a single one of them would apply for the job, but the job in terms of keeping the department going would not miss a beat. That is energizing and renourishing of my soul every single day.

Probably my most satisfying experience in the early years was when I hired my very first nurse. When I first took over, the staff was there. Some of them had trained me, and some I had worked with as peers. The very first nurse I interviewed, I chose, I hired, and I mentored. I realized the fact that I was actually shaping [new nurses'] futures. They were just starting out. This was their very first job. They had no preconceived notion. They didn't know what to expect. I helped guide them and helped show them what nursing was really like here at this hospital as well as in the community in general.

They Offer Opportunities for Autonomy and Freedom

This aspect of generativity involves the pleasure of passing on and "offering up" what the individual has built by gifting a next generation with respect, power, and autonomy (Bradley & James, 1998; McAdams, Hart, & Maruna, 1998). Managers frequently conveyed the goal of training their staff to be independent of them. In the following examples, nurse managers have a wonderful way of explaining their sense of confidently handing their kids the keys to the car.

Examples from Interviews

I have—not alone, of course, but with the help of the staff—I think I've cultivated an environment where I don't have to be there all the time. I know that if I need to leave or if I'm going to be gone for a bit of time that the floor will still run efficiently. The staff is just an extension of me. I don't feel like everything just goes to heck when I'm not there. Honestly, I do not even think twice that if I'm not going to be there that they are not going to be overstaffed or slacking off, not at all. But again, that comes from not pushing down their throats. It's really from giving them the autonomy and giving them respect and letting them be professional. That makes them want to do a professional job.

> [My mentor's] goal was to make sure that everybody was competent enough to work without her, and that is my goal. I have gone from one CN4 to six in my leadership growth. I remember when I first went away and I was hysterical the whole week I was gone. Now, I take the phone off. I go and they are here, and I know it's going to be here when I come back. Yes, because they need [that confidence,] too. What happens if I'm in a car accident tomorrow? They need to survive; the patients need to do well. For me, if I don't do that, I am sending them out to fail.

ARDOR

"Call me corny," warned a nurse manager at a meeting in Boston, "but I have been in the same job for 25 years, and I still really love my job and the people I

- **Cherishes relationships**
- **Invests in patient care**
- **Commits to organization**

work with." His comment mirrored one of the striking aspects of the NMEP data: the depth and breadth of passion expressed.

In the NMEP, managers frequently used the word "love" ("I love working here"; "I love taking care of patients"; "I love working with these nurses") and chose superlative adjectives ("amazing," "phenomenal," "wows me with their skills"). They spoke of devotion and calling to their work ("They recognize that nursing is not what I do. It is not a profession; it is who I am.").

The growing literature on work engagement (Wagner & Harter, 2006) links it to passion about the job (Borchardt, 2005; Cortes, 2004; Gubman, 2004) and a heightened emotional connection to work and organization that goes beyond job satisfaction. The numerous examples of intensity of feeling in managers from five of the six organizations in the NMEP evoked the notion of "ardor," which is defined by warmth, animation, and excitement. Clearly, this element of ardor drives nurse managers' continued LOS to the purpose of their work. It can be tracked in three distinct areas.

They Cherish Great Relationships with Staff, Colleagues, and Leadership

Managers' descriptions of strong relationships and bonds throughout the organization echo Mycek's (1998) suggestion that health care is about the business of relationships. One nurse manager offered an anatomy of her ardor: "We have a great staff. [It's] the people who make a difference to me every single day, and it's my relationship with the medical team, with my boss, with [CNO's name], with the woman at the cafeteria who I buy my coffee from in the morning—that is what makes me want to be here every day."

Examples from Interviews

I cannot begin to explain to you how energized I am every morning when I come in because I will be working with this group. I am so happy that we have transformed not just the environment, but also the people. I have seen the change, the 60% who stayed with me after the changes. . . . No matter which department you go to, they will tell you, "Those are the best nurses in the building; they are the most customer service oriented." I am so proud. I could go anywhere and double my salary maybe, but I don't think I could form or nurture another group as well as we have nurtured each other here so that I would be as happy in any other setting.

It comes right back to the staff. I have just an amazing group of people to work with. Watching the staff work through those situations and then basically coming out on the other end with a positive outcome—those are the things that fire me up. We had this very tragic little girl the other day, just a horrendous health history, and she probably won't survive for a very long time. Watching one of my nurses who is a guy and has got a family and teenage daughters—watching him hold this little girl, I'm mean we're all like just choked up sitting here, and how he just loved on this little girl while she was here in this really scary environment, a very painful environment. Seeing those kinds of things and just knowing the kind of people I'm surrounded by, those are the things that fire me up.

The confidence and the skill of these nurses are phenomenal; they are so good . . . doctors fight to get their patients on my floor because of the skills that these nurses have. It overwhelms me. I feel so honored to work with such a gifted group of people, and that continues to just be the driving force. It's knowing when I'm not there, they do cartwheels over anything that needs to be done. This continually happens time and time again. I was just on vacation last week. I came back today and at least ten different people said, "Your group was just phenomenal last week." It constantly wows me on their skills.

They Are Deeply Invested in Patient Care

To listen to engaged nurse managers is to witness the marriage of Myeck's (1998) business of relationships with the focus on mission (Girard, Linton, & Bestner, 2005). Here is a manager describing her investment: "Sometimes you don't recognize [the patients], bless their little hearts, when they come back with hair, but their hearts speak to them. They end up in the right place, and for me that does not grow old, it doesn't grow old."

Examples from Interviews

> I can see it in my staff. I see it in the stories that they tell me, the situations that I know of, hear of from multiple different places and either seek out additional information or get it just in its own little nutshell. It's just a thing of beauty where the best caring and the most personal care happened for somebody right when they needed it. In a lot of ways, I don't know what could be better. We have clinical specialties where there are lots of opportunities . . . for sensitivity, for caring for people who are incredibly vulnerable. The honor when I see people provide nursing care is amazing.

> There are countless patient stories that are just phenomenal that if I sit and think about it, I often cry. It's amazing how we deal with the surgical oncology population, who are often our age. I'll walk past the room and I'll see a nurse just sitting there, holding a patient's hand, and just talking and asking her, "Go ahead and tell me about how you are feeling and what does it mean, when you say you are going to call your husband and tell him that you are dying." It's just amazing. It's amazing because even with all the technology, all the medicines, all the procedures, it still comes down to sitting at that bedside, holding someone's hand when they are in their lowest moment. I see that on a daily basis.

> [I often] get a "thank you" note about a patient who has passed away from their family, saying what a difference the staff made in their last three weeks of their life. . . . I can go on and on because that happens all the time, and it's because of the people I work with; it's what they do and they do it so well. They are an amazing, amazing group of people. When people talk about my units, I am overwhelmed with pride for that. When I talk about what I do and the people I work with, it stirs the passion that I have in nursing and [reminds me] how important it is to me.

They Are Deeply Committed to Their Organization

Commitment to the organization is at the core of employee engagement (Wagner & Harter, 2006). The depth of gratitude and admiration in the data conveys an enduring sense of connection for nurse managers. One manager elaborated, "I just love this hospital. I would not want to work in any other facility. I think every learning opportunity you want is here. You are recognized as individuals and not numbers."

Examples from Interviews

> I just cannot believe what [this organization] has given to me. It has nurtured me to grow. What I have given is very minimal compared to what it has given to me.

... We have patients who are dying and I worked with them and with the sisters [nuns], and it was "What do you need? We need to support you." You should have seen that; they run around and get all the stuff that people need. I have started to remember, and I always want to cry when I remember. It's integrity with respect and wisdom.

They are not doing it because someone else is watching; they are not doing it for a lot of reasons that might be a motivator that is less than true. It's true; it's about compassion and caring and just seeing. I overhear small snippets as I walk in the halls. I can see in the way someone who comes back to us is received at the front desk. It's just incredibly touching. It's really moving; it fills me. Those are the moments when I know this is exactly what I want. I'm not here by accident. This is a perfect fit and I would have to say, what else can I hope for than a place where I can see this type of human compassion in action?

IDENTIFICATION

A nurse manager from Cincinnati described what she finds gratifying about her work: "Everything we do affects patient care, from the design of our new units, to keeping them clean on a day-to-day basis. Even though I

- **Sees own achievement in the success of staff**
- **Maintains a link to direct patient care**
- **Creates an atmosphere for superb care**

don't do 'hands-on' care for our patients, they are the focus of everything we do every day."

Management mavens are fond of the truism that a manager is someone who gets his or her work done through other people. Nurse managers who want to nurture their own engagement, like the one from Cincinnati, must take matters one step further. My discussions, classes, and interviews with nurse managers suggest that seeing their own achievement (by identifying with the work of others) is critical in their engagement as a nurse manager.

For the nurse manager, whose former bedside patient care has been replaced with managerial tasks and goals, *identification* seems to compensate for the loss of, or lessening of direct patient care. Keeping a clear LOS with the care at the bedside via their staff enables managers to stay in contact with the care-taking focus that initially attracted them to nursing.

Contemporary psychologists have expanded Freud's (1933) definition of identification to describe it as a person's positive association with—or assumption of—the qualities, characteristics, or views of another person or group without losing their own identity (Silverman, 2002; Valliant, 1993). It is the incorporation of positive aspects of your experience into your sense of who you are. Nurse leader Ti King (1999) describes this signature element in terms of working through people to enhance the nurse manager's own growth, potential, and accomplishments.

Three themes in the NMEP interview data underlined engaged managers' capacity to identify with the work of their staff and organization—as if it were their own. These themes have been expanded in my continuing conversations, classes, and in e-mails from nurse managers.

They Describe and Enjoy Their Part in the Success and Accomplishments of Their Staff

Psychologist Charles Tart (1975) calls this aspect of identification "this is me." Managers seem to enhance their engagement by naming their contribution to patient care and staff development. "Everything that I get pride out of comes from the floor and how it runs," one manager wrote of the gratification she obtained from her staff's safety record. She also noted, "I helped make their job easier and more efficient."

Examples from Interviews

> I love when I get reports back that show high patient satisfaction. That is always gratifying for me and also when they recognize the nursing staff. Their success is my success. If my fall program and medication reconciliation program were 100% compliant, that would be very satisfying for me.

> The very first thing that comes to mind is my staff. We keep getting [recognitions] such as "best patient satisfaction in the medical center." That is my staff. That is my staff working with the patients, and that makes me feel very proud. They are doing an awesome job of taking care of patients. I am leading them to do that. I have hired them all. We work together as a team.

They Maintain a Link to the Care of the Patient at the Bedside

Studies of nurse satisfaction (Bunsey, DeFazio, & Jones, 1991; Fletcher, 2001) have underlined the importance of patient care activities as making a difference in the life of a patient. The NMEP data suggest that linking management activity to the end result of patient care is critical for long-term engagement. A manager explained her LOS by saying, "I was able to stay in the [nurse manager] position because I thought of the position as a way of making sure the people were taken care of the way I'd want them to be taken care of."

Examples from Interviews

> I used to think that I should really go back to bedside nursing. In bedside nursing, you can affect your assignment of patients for a day. As a manager, I affect 52 staff people. To me, the influence in terms of giving is much more, and I can have much more of an input, for better or worse—hopefully for better.
>
> It's making a difference in a way that is maybe not so directly tied to patients as far as caring for patients but knowing that what I do in so many other ways, it makes a difference for patients and families and for the staff that I work with.

They Create an Atmosphere Where Staff Can Provide Superb Patient Care
Ti King (1999) calls this aspect "provoking leadership," and Kouzes and Posner (2003) refer to "enabling others to act." Nurse managers offered numerous examples of giving staff support, responsibility, and visibility. Two examples: "If I can develop my staff to be able to take good care of the patients, then I am perfectly satisfied" and "To know that our patients are having an extraordinary experience, to be involved in processes that facilitate this and to know that my staff has contributed."

Examples from Interviews

> I see my responsibility as also creating a healing environment for all the staff that work here, so that they are taking care of themselves in a way that they are then energized and have what they need to take care of patients and families and give their best.
>
> [Showing a poster:] This is something by Henry David Thoreau; it says, "It is something to able to paint a picture or to carve a statue and so we make a few objects beautiful, but it is far more glorious to carve and paint the atmosphere in which we work to affect the quality of the day that this is the highest we are." . . . Well, creating an environment where people feel so empowered and positive and capable . . . translates into how they interact with the patients.

EYES ON THE PRIZE
Last week, I assigned a group of 30 AONE nurse manager fellows, who were sitting at tables of five, to build the tallest possible structure with the items that were on their table. The prize, voted by the class and awarded in chocolate coins, went to the group who built a sculpture of water glasses and notebooks.

As the class restored the room to its pre-game order, we all agreed that when you are building a tower, it is easy to keep an eye on your goal. But for managers, who were drawn to nursing out of the desire to care for the patient at the bedside, the biggest challenge is maintaining a line of sight to that purpose.

Dozens of examples in this chapter map line of sight in the crucial signatures of *mission primacy, identification, ardor,* and *generativity.* For nurse managers, this could mean doing the math of how many more patients they can serve as a manager, expressing pride in their staff nurse posse, speaking valentines about their team or patients, or growing ducks in their own image. In every example, we see the work of nurses who have translated their devotion to patient care into the thoughts, words, and deeds of a manager.

The alignment with purpose is one of the two crucibles of nurse manager engagement. The other is emotional mastery, which is defined by six signature behaviors that allow managers to meet the unique emotional challenges of being in charge.

CHAPTER 3

The Signature Behaviors of Emotional Mastery

Interviews with nurses about the unique emotional demands of management bring to mind Sternberg's (1997) definition of practical intelligence: knowing what to say to whom, knowing when to say it, and knowing how to say it for maximum effect. This kind of emotional mastery is captured in the story of Norma B., an emergency room (ER) manager trained to make quick decisions who moved from one coast to another: "I came with an East Coast management style in terms of making decisions and I discovered here that was not the case." As she explained:

> The communication here was not only that you had to be very careful in how you spoke, but what your face looked like, what you did with your hands, how fast you made an answer. I got tremendous resistance in the beginning. I was perceived as abrupt, rash, disrespectful, for things that I was oblivious to. One of the things that didn't happen that made it hard, but for me humility then made the success, was trying to learn to maintain my standards that I feel very, very strongly about. I am very ethically grounded . . . very, very patient care-oriented. I didn't care if I hurt your feelings if it was going to save a patient. I had to learn how not to sacrifice that, but get the message across in a different way.

Over a period of several years, Norma developed several facets of emotional mastery. She learned, as she put it, "to be massaged and manipulated within myself, to be able to be comfortable with my own skin, keep my standards, and yet deliver the message with a manner that could be accepted."

Six elements of emotional mastery have been linked with engagement: boundary clarity, reflection, self-regulation, attunement, change agility, and an affirmative framework. Each element has the potential to enrich a manager's longevity and performance.

BOUNDARY CLARITY

A nurse manager in San Francisco explained boundary clarity as important to the initiation and long-term sustainment of a nurse manager: "I was a nurse for 15 years on this unit. Those staff members who were my friends were no longer. To succeed as a manager, you must be consistent and fair and do what is right for your patient."

- **Models and displays appropriate boundaries**
- **Builds strong internal boundaries**
- **Creates emotional insulation**
- **Connects with others without losing a sense of self**

The frequent use of the phrase "not taking it personally" in interviews and conversations with managers indicated their marked preference for creating, maintaining, and restoring clear boundaries between self and others (Adams, 2005; Hartmann, 1991). Boundary clarity, defined as the capacity to build strong connections with others without losing sense of self, is a key to emotional mastery for nurse managers. It can be discerned among nurse managers in three distinct ways.

They Model and Display Appropriate Boundaries

Helping nurse managers set realistic boundaries has been linked to creating healthcare cultures of retention (Manion, 2005). The nurse managers in the NMEP study, especially those promoted from within, have made a clear transition between nurse peer and nurse manager who is responsible for outcome. "You need to separate yourself a bit," warned one manager.

Examples from Interviews

> One of my RNs just got blasted by a night-shift nurse one time; I mean, it was devastating to her. She ended up going to counseling later. . . . It just drove me crazy. [I told my nurse] that I just thought this is a reflection on [the night nurse] and where she's at in her work. And if she's attacking you personally, it's still about her. . . . [So] I say in work language, "She has a performance issue," just to use some of those words, and we're going to help her with that, and she's having problems communicating her feelings without becoming personal. I just think in some ways if you can rephrase it, you can see it for what it is. It's work; it's a professional situation.

> Very simply, [I do not] take things personally. If somebody had plans to leave very soon after being oriented, or perhaps wasn't that upfront about their call-ins or whatever, I took all that really personally at first. I think part of that was because I hadn't learned; I still thought of myself as one of the staff. Not that I don't think that now, but I realize that you do have to separate yourself a little bit from the staff in order to make unbiased judgments, in order to make calls that are correct.

> You can't just be one of their buddies. I was their peer, and I still think of myself as their peer, but I needed to separate myself a little bit.

They Build Strong Internal Boundaries

Hartmann (1991) used the term "thick boundaries" to characterize those individuals who are able to maintain their focus and equilibrium in the face of the strong feelings of others. The phrase "they were not attacking *me*" was a frequent indicator of the capacity of nurse managers to separate their own thoughts and feelings from those of others.

Examples from Interviews

> There is a gap of the intensity that isn't mine personally, but it is my staff's. Being able to translate that and be an ambassador of sorts—this is really what it means; it means that I need to be able to communicate that effectively.

> If things aren't going well in your personal life, your way to deal with that sometimes is being angry with everything at work, or being an excellent clinical provider at this point. I think it depends on being able to figure out what is the real thing that they are angry about . . . trying to figure out the root of what people are talking about.

> With staff, a lot of times I found out at the end when I did take it personally, they really weren't mad—*it was not a personal attack*. It was just, "I'm angry about this scenario." There were times that the decision I made did affect them. I can think of a very clear one: I wanted to do scheduling the way I did it when I was a staff nurse where I worked. I learned through that, personally [they were not] attacking me—it was the idea that they had to work Christmas.

They Can Create Emotional Insulation

Nurse managers are adept at building what psychiatrist Louis Ormond (1994) called a healthy "insulation barrier." This kind of internal boundary allows experience in, but protects the self from being overwhelmed by negative emotions in self or others. This healthy process is captured in the comment, "If I took it as a personal attack, I would never survive."

Examples from Interviews

> Not taking things personally when people are upset—I think that was one of the hardest things for me in the beginning. If I could not get over that, I would have never stayed in the role. Because if you take every negative thing people have to

say about the unit or what's going on, [if] you take it as a personal attack on you, I would have never survived. I have come a long way in that aspect.

I had a nurse who needed a lot of changes in the schedule, had a lot of personal issues, and maybe three months later, [the nurse] decided . . . to work somewhere else. I was very upset. I thought, "How dare you do that to me? I bent over backward for you; I have really gone out of my way for you." I didn't say it like that, but I definitely was upset and probably let [the nurse] know. Again, this was probably not the correct response either, but I think I taught myself (a) I can't take it personally and (b) [the nurse] didn't do this to me. If I choose to react this way to it, that's my issue. I chose to bend over backward for [the nurse,] and again [that was] my issue. I had to make sure that I could only give what I thought was acceptable and not expect allegiance forever and forever. . . . [First,] I can only do things that are in my control; I can't control someone else's behavior. . . . [Second,] I better not do any more than what I want to do if it puts me in the arena of expecting something back for it. I'll do it because it makes sense or it's the right thing to do. It may or may not get the desired outcome.

They Restore Clear Boundaries and Perspective Through Disengagement

A manager described the act of making boundaries in this way: "I try to step back and let the person get all of their emotions out. Then, I try to explain to them and to myself where they are coming from and where I am coming from and what I'm trying to achieve. I try to find the middle ground." Heifeitz and Linksky (2002) labeled such acts of deliberate detachment and disengagement from heated situations—in an attempt to review the problem—as "getting off the dance floor and up on the balcony." Managers' capacity to stand back and assess problems was a strong pattern in the NMEP data.

Examples from Interviews

I needed to, when things were happening, to step back and say, "They're not doing this to me. . . . [F]or whatever reason, they've chosen to present this way, to act this way. I can't take it personally." It was really upsetting to me at first, and then I realized I needed to stop and take a moment and realize that whatever they needed to do was their own issue and not directly related to me.

There are times when family members are just adamant. What I try to do is bring them into my office and remove them from the audience and see what the real problem is. Nine times out of ten, it has nothing to do with whatever they are screaming about. I try to see what is underneath the emotions.

I try to make whatever the subject is number one. I'll tell staff, "You are not bad people. You may have made a bad decision, but that does not make you a bad person." And in doing that, that takes away sometimes the harshness, but still drives home what you are trying to get at, or to make your point. Even when I talk with physicians, if I try to really pose [this kind of question,] and often I do, it's because Ms. Smith in this room is having this difficult time with me—not because I want you to make my job easier or whatever. I take away that personal piece of it and try to put out the facts of the subject.

REFLECTION

The capacity of engaged nurse managers for self-appraisal through reflecting and learning from experience was a dominant theme. Their responses suggested the postmodern proverb: Call it research rather than failure. For many

- **Leverages lessons from experience**
- **Scans for cues about self and others in the workplace**
- **Observes the effect of the manager's behavior on others**

managers, reflection is flavored with self-forgiveness and learning through the experience of doing things wrong.

For example, one manager in the NMEP study spoke with unflinching honesty about a staff survey and her responses to it:

The staff had some very cruel and very pointed negative things to say. One portion was about me, about my leadership style. I've learned a lot of things since then about it. A lot of people saw the results of what people thought of me, and they weren't pretty. I had to take a very close look at myself. So for the last year and a half, in a sense, even though I feel very good about a number of things that I am capable of doing, there is a piece that has continued to be held over my neck in terms of fixing those nuances, and remembering at all times to do something a little bit different. Well, the most recent survey results showed such a significant improvement at my 360[-degree] feedback that my own director gave me just yesterday, where staff were allowed to make free-flowing comments—they showed that even at this stage of my development, I have still made such a further leap in improving my communication and my ability to lead this department that I now finally have the sword buried. But I don't forget the sword; I am very cognizant of never forgetting it.

Three facets of reflection are critical to engaged nurse managers.

They Leverage Lessons from Experience

Learning from experience is a central tenet of nursing education (Burnard, 1992; Edmondson, 1996, 1999) and has been a focus of the literature of reflective practice (Charalambous, 2003; John, 2004; John & Freshwater, 1996; Schon, 1987). Mackoff and Wenet (2004) referred to the capacity to leverage lessons from relationships and experiences as central to the development of leadership because it uncovers important information and drives the opportunity for course correction or continuation.

Examples from Interviews

> We learn by mistake and by error. When I look back, I say, "Those are valuable lessons for me, because that is what built me up to what I am today." You learn from small steps, and then all the way up. You gather everything all together, and you put it in your notebook. When you go back and study it, you can say, "Oh, yeah, I should have done differently here or I could have been better." Or sometimes, "I'm really proud of myself that I was able to do this." What I learned from that experience is that you don't have to know everything to lead. You just have to learn a lot of that. But you need to have commitment, motivation, and patience to go along with that. Once in a while, when I take on some task, I say, "Oh, my gosh, I don't know if I'm able to do it." I always go back to that time. I didn't know anything but I did it.
>
> I made a lot of mistakes, so I had to learn a lot of hard lessons. I think the most important lesson that I learned, and I learned early on, was dealing fairly and effectively with problem staff. I had a nursing attendant who put a nurse's license in jeopardy, and she did not lose her position. They said, "Show me the documentation that said that you told her this specific thing to do in this situation." I couldn't do that. That was a hard lesson for me. That was a lesson in terms of, how I do overlook people? How do I document that orientation?

They Scan for Clues About Self and Others

Nurse Leader Ti Hill (1997) has emphasized the importance of the ability to scan for relevant cues about self and others in workplace situations—and then to reflect on, and make sense of, these cues. This is another element of reflective practice (John & Freshwater, 1996). It is a kind of anthropology of the self, where managers are both participants and observers at the same time.

For one manager, scanning means "watching how people get things done and picking up cues." For another, it means "I learned how to be politically savvy when I speak to different people. I learned a little of what I call the schmooze factor."

Examples from Interviews

> [I have learned to] identify a physical cue that preceded a poor communication style. I have learned . . . to recognize what my communication style was when I was

impassioned about something and when I was becoming irrational, so that often I have a mantra that I say to myself. It's two different mantras. One is "slow down your speech and lower your voice." It forces me to speak and think slower when I speak because my mind is processing so fast. As fast as I process, I tend to give the impression that "what you have to say is not important because I've already gotten to the solution. I have already skipped over all of your input." That might not be the case, but I have to make myself slow down so that what you are seeing from me is that engagement, that active listening.

They Observe Their Own Behavior and Its Impact on Others

Behavioral economist John Adams (2005) called this process becoming the "impartial spectator" and "the eye of the third person." Mackoff and Wenet (2004) have detailed how leaders' knowledge of their own thoughts and reactions enables them to gauge their effect on others. A manager further defined self-appraisal in practical terms: "It's self-awareness and being careful that I don't lose people working with me."

Examples from Interviews

Part of it is a self-check. Part of it is being able to learn and to use my peers—witnesses to [whom I can] say, "That is not where I wanted to go. Did you see where it got off track? I'm not sure what I said." I want to own my part and . . . have the outcome be more important than me.

I have to be careful that I stay politically correct but still get things done. If something really bothers me, I have to be careful that I'm not too "big mouth" . . . just making sure I don't end up looking like a troublemaker by always bringing out the problems that are around. I'm advocating for what is best . . . I think just being careful how I say things, so I won't look like a complainer.

My nature was, and still is to an extent, when my staff are in the hall and at a computer, I don't interrupt them to say, "Hello, how's your day going?" because they get interrupted all the time. I don't want to be a source of interruption. That could be received as someone who doesn't care. Well, I care, but I am not going to interrupt you. So I just talk about that now. My learning from that was okay, it's possible to be misunderstood. I don't like to be misunderstood; it really bugs me, so I will take whatever time it takes to clarify what I meant. I may need to be more forward—then that's what I do differently from that earlier learning. I let people know how I work. There are some times when I literally walk on to the unit and I just hope to get back to my office with all the things still in my head so I can actually do something about them. I don't have a good poker face necessarily."

SELF-REGULATION

Nurse managers in the NMEP study and in a variety of settings find it easy to define self-regulation and to express its practice as a hard-learned lesson.

- **Practices restraint**
- **Responds rather than reacts**
- **Perseveres with patience**

One pithy definition: "I have learned not to knee-jerk respond." This capacity to manage one's internal emotional states is critical to personal competence (Goleman, 1998b; Salovey & Mayer, 1990, 1997). These behaviors are also a facet of "emotional labor" (Grandey, 2000; Vitello-Cicciu, 2003), which involves regulating thoughts, feelings, and speech to achieve organizational goals or expectations.

Nurse managers repeatedly used the word patience to detail three distinct aspects of self-regulation. As a manager from Maui explained, "I have learned patience—to listen and observe and to time when to broach the subject of change. I have learned to change in small increments, so as not to overwhelm."

They Use Restraint to Keep Emotions and Impulses in Check

Whether they are dealing with a patient with charisma bypass surgery or an angry staff nurse, engaged nurse managers employ restraint. For them, this element of self-control involves keeping emotions and impulses in check as well as conserving energy and resources by choosing battles wisely (Goleman, 1995; Zillman, 1993). A manager wryly observed, "Sometimes it is learning when *not* to say something."

Examples from Interviews

> I think one of the most important things that I have learned is to control my own affect when I'm angry or if I'm impatient. If I'm angry with a staff member, I don't want them to know that. I do not want them to know. Now, that doesn't mean that I can't say, "I'm very frustrated with your behavior." I just don't mean my facial expression; I mean my emotions. Because when you get emotional, you lose your objectivity. You say things that you regret. You don't do a good job at it, and I think that to be a good manager and a good leader, you really need to maintain your objectivity in very charged situations.

> If somebody insults me or whatever, I have to tell myself, "Do not speak." And it's not even expression. When I [have felt] myself welling up inside—because I have spoken in that emotional state so many times—it just blew [up] in my face. Nothing horrible happened. But my effectiveness as a leader, no matter what the content was that I was saying, was compromised because of the tone. So, if somebody does something, a staff member does something, and I just feel a physical, emotional state, that's my cue to say, "Nobody's dying here; this can wait."

I have learned to choose my battles and not to choose losing battles. If you know you are going to lose the battle, don't waste your time fighting it. I [have] learned to be as cooperative as I can be. Maybe what I want is not necessarily the plan. We were in a cluster concept, so there was a lot of cooperation that was desirable at the time and it wasn't always forthcoming. In order to gain that cooperation from all of the different pieces of the cluster, sometimes I had to give up things that I thought I wanted for the greater good. I can have such an impact on [the situation], even though it's not what I choose, but I think I can turn the situation into something that is good for the hospital and for me and for my nursing staff.

They Respond—Rather Than Just React

Suspending judgment—that is, thinking before acting—is a key to self-regulation (Goleman, 1998a). Nurse managers often labeled this as another facet of patience that they accomplished through their deliberate slowing down of reaction time and in-depth listening: "You need to take it all in, before you react to situations."

Examples from Interviews

It often means listening differently, asking questions, not arriving at a judgment without enough information. [It means] really being open to that particular human being and their take on it, even though I'm thinking, "Gee whiz, what happened? How did it get there?", but to not to allow them the opportunity to read my internal bubble. To really make sure that I get it and understand what they were doing— that's part of the patience. [It means] really being able to take a deep breath and say, "Tell me more; I don't quite understand."

Yes, I think listening is a form of patience. I think maybe some of the techniques which I have done with some people who react quickly are to take ten deep breaths before saying anything and follow through by saying, "Tell me more." It's a way of buying time so that you are not reacting. If it is a nurse, I will say, "Tell me more about what happened." If it is a patient or family member, [I will just listen] to what they have to say about that. Sometimes I can't do anything about it, and sometimes I agree with them.

I had a family member who was very hostile to one of our staff members. When I walked on the unit, the staff was ready to go into the room and protect their peers and tell [the family member] that wasn't right. I explained to them that we don't want to add flame to the fire; we want to take a deep breath. Let me go in there and I can . . . explain the situation to [the family] and also nicely let them know it's not acceptable to treat people or staff that way. The staff wanted to immediately go in, but I told them to step back and try to see why [the family member] was upset and that we needed to go back in the room and explain what was going on. I was able to be patient with the family member even though the behavior was not right.

They Practice Perseverance

There is a brand of perseverance, as practiced by engaged nurse managers, that is equal parts patience, tenacity, and forbearance. It is also linked to the ability to manage emotions (Salovey & Mayer, 1990) and to the use of self-regulation to meet organizational goals (Grandey, 2000). There were many variations on this theme: "I can be incredibly patient. I can repeat myself a hundred different ways if that's what's required."

Humor was often enlisted in the description of perseverance and patience. Here is one manager's wry observation: "We have to have realistic expectations and know how to stay patient—how to keep your eye on the ball, but learn how almost nothing happens immediately. If it happens immediately, it's because a code light went off, not really ever because it's a management code."

Examples from Interviews

A tremendous amount of patience is knowing that there are things that have been in place in an organization for a long period of time and they're not necessarily going to be open to new ideas right off the bat. [The key is to be] able to begin to plant the seed of ideas and just sort of [cultivate] that seed over a period of time—then either it becomes a standard of practice over time just because it's been slowly working in, or it becomes somebody else's idea. And then it ultimately works out anyway.

We do a lot of space planning here in ambulatory; we move clinics all the time, back and forth. I was actually having a discussion with the sign man, and it was really getting challenging. And I kept smiling and kept smiling and saying, "You know these are the reasons we should be doing it." And so I just kept saying that these are the reasons and my colleague says to me, "How can you have said that with a smile, over and over and over?" I said, "Because I had to. That was the only way that I was going to win."

ATTUNEMENT

When asked about the strengths she brings to her management role, a TCAB nurse manager in San Francisco gave a heartfelt definition of attunement (Mackoff & Wenet, 2004): "My philosophy is to treat everyone with the greatest respect, from the housekeeper to the VP." Her comment suggests attunement is a powerful hybrid of the capacity to appreciate the uniqueness of others and

- Displays regard for individual contributions
- Understands diverse perspectives
- Sets aside assumptions to learn from others

the ability to take on their perspective—even when it is different from your own view. Nurse managers spoke of three distinct aspects of this strength.

They Show Regard for Individual Contributions

Mackoff and Wenet (2004) have described the capacity of leaders to regard and prize the lives and contributions of individual staff members and colleagues. Buckingham (2005) reports that the recognition of the unique strengths of staff members is critical to employee engagement. For many nurse managers, attunement is infused with ardor: "I work with fabulous people who are resourceful and brilliant care providers."

Examples from Interviews

[It is] knowing that each individual brings something different to the department. [It is recognizing] whatever their gifts are or whatever their challenges are, and then working through those with each individual. Probably one of my biggest challenges is that I tend in some ways to try to work through problems with an individual almost too long at times. It's almost to a fault in a sense that, if I have somebody that I really see an opportunity in and I think that person will eventually come around, will grow, will mature, into what we hope they would be as an employee as well as a person, I will work with them and work with them and work with them. We have a very culturally diverse group in our department, and it's really kind of fun to watch how those people interact with one another as well as how they interact with patients.

I remember little things. It allows me, I think, to manage people if there's something going on. Like I know, for instance, [suppose] there's something not right with one of my nursing assistants. Well, you know what—she's got a sister who's in the ICU intubated and is on life support. [This kind of information] helps me to know that [why the nurse is] not performing to the best that she normally does, instead of judging her for [being] lazy.

They Seek to Understand Diverse Viewpoints and Perspectives

The capacity to take another point of view—to stand in someone else's shoes—has long been considered the milestone in cognitive development (Piaget, 1983) and social competence (Galinsky & Moskowitz, 2000). It has been called "perspective taking" (Selman, 1980) and "empathic accuracy" (Ickes, 1997). One engaged nurse manager explained this ability in the context of management by saying, "It really forced me to be open minded. You see different kinds of people [who are different from me] and it gives you an appreciation for diversity."

Examples from Interviews

> To really understand what the other person is thinking and feeling and to really go there with that other person. That "you get it" kind of thing, and the person knows you get it; [then] that the person knows that I am totally getting it and that I am listening to them. When staff [nurses] come to me individually about their private issues and I listen to them, I want them to know that I totally get it and I am there for them. Sometimes I cannot give them every single request they have, but I do get it. If I can't do it at that time, it's not that I don't understand, but it's that I just can't.

> I never forgot what my first days [as a staff nurse] were like, so I always felt like I knew what the nurses needed and what the staff needed, and I wasn't shy about jumping in and just helping them. And that's really what they needed because they were just starting out—never forget that. This is part of empathy. [Recalls her mother's illness.] I think it just goes back to [the fact that] I haven't lost that sense of what the nurse wants and needs at the bedside. That's what, if you don't forget that, [if] you can keep that in mind, you can satisfy your staff. I just kept thinking, well, what would make me happy and not forgetting, like I said, those first days. And then just from a patient and staff perspective, [from a] patient and family perspective, [what is important] in terms of trying to make them satisfied.

They Set Aside Their Own Assumptions to Get The Whole Story

Mackoff and Wenet (2004) referred to this aspect of attunement as getting "the whole story." The philosopher Husserl (1999) originated the term "bracketing" to describe the process of setting aside your viewpoint. It is an element of emotional mastery that psychologist Robert Kegan (1983) calls "learning about a reality quite different from my own." Many nurse managers accomplish this with a variation on the intention of "always getting their side of the story before I go jumping to conclusions."

Examples from Interviews

> Beth was the night director of nursing at the time, and she always said there were two sides to every story. If there was a staff conflict or patient/family conflict, we needed to hear both sides before we could intervene in the situation. On [night shifts] that was certainly true, but in the day shift with all the physicians and families and everything else, I think that is one of the things I always remember—to step back and listen to both sides before you offer some kind of solution. I think it's very important when family members are complaining about staff to hear what the staff have to say. A lot of times it's quite the opposite.

> When someone is complaining about someone and I would say, "Thank you very much for letting me know. There are always two sides of the coin, and I am going

to call this person. I want to hear her side, but after I have heard her side, I would like to bring both of you into my office so that we can straighten this out." The first time they heard me say that, it made them feel like they needed to be prepared. I would tell them, "I will get back to you, but I have to hear both sides because [the other person is] not here to defend her side." And I called the other person and I played it that I had heard some concerns about something that happened last Tuesday and she tells me her side. So I listen and then I tell her, "Can we bring somebody in so that we can straighten this out?" I bring in the third person and say, "Whatever happens in this room will not go out."

CHANGE AGILITY

A 20-year nurse manager from Columbus, Indiana, revealed her change agility when she wrote, "It is important to remain curious, be open

- **Challenges the process**
- **Welcomes and originates change**
- **Seeks change through new learning**

to change, be flexible and agile—and be willing to forgive self and others—due to the ever-changing world of health care."

The themes and variations on mastering change that were brought up in the study interviews, and in my many meetings with nurse managers, evoked Chris Musselwhite's (2005) phrase "change agility." They also provided examples of the kind of transformative leadership behaviors and attitudes that drive and model change (Marszalek, Gaucher, & Coffey, 1991; McGuire & Kennedy, 2006). Three aspects of this individual signature element in engaged nurse managers can be detailed.

They Challenge the Process

Agile nurse managers are the unit fixers, the first to describe a problem, the first to volunteer to work on a solution. Kouzes and Posner (2003) identified this capacity to challenge the process as a key leadership practice. It includes questioning the status quo and promoting innovation, growth, and improvement.

Examples from Interviews

I think it's the ability for me sometimes to even take units that aren't as high functioning [and to] turn them into a place where people are proud of where they work. If there are derogatory statements made about them, I can sit there and say, "Do you like being called that?'" I said, "With the kind of people that you are and the hard work that you do, how do you feel when you hear yourself refer to this unit?" They all kind of looked at me and said, "We don't like it." I said, "Well, then, we are going to change it because that is not the reputation you want." I've done that. The people who I work with and how they respond and how I respond to them—that's what keeps me being a manager for so long, and it's exciting to me.

There were apparently some issues with that manager, so they asked me if I would take on the dual role of manager and clinical specialist and [manage] the first unit to do patient-focused care. That is really why I took [the job]—because it was a huge change process and I loved that. It was because I saw the possibilities for what we could do [and] because we had made such strides forward. I am always going on to the next step, I think. I do change the processes pretty well. We have done projects in orthopedics always, and I am usually the first to try something, because I do that well with the staff and corporate staff and make them want to do it.

They Welcome and Originate Change

Engaged nurse managers don't just cope with change, they are energized by it. Musselwhite (1995) used the word "originators" to characterize those who welcome and seek dramatic change. Data from nurse managers suggest that these originators are also skilled in coping with ambiguity and approaching novel situations and ideas (Goleman, 1998a, 1998b). This brand of change agility is reflected in the comment, "When things get too comfortable, I start looking for something else."

Examples from Interviews

If I didn't learn, I think it would be very disappointing and boring. I'm always given the chance for new opportunity. There is always a class or conference I can go to. I have had several different management jobs within this level of management, and what [kept] me going is that each job was a little bit different. It was a little bit of a "fix it" kind of thing. With the current job that I have now, which has [lasted] for a year and a half, there were also many issues with this unit. What keeps me [interested] is that each job is a little different.

I could see in staff meetings when I introduced myself and said a few things about myself, I could tell the whole energy was so negative in the beginning. I could see it in their faces. Even in the nurses, there was no connection, there was no eye contact. It was sort of forlorn and withdrawn. After a short period of time, I got them energized and let them know they were important and they were terrific. . . . When I worked as a staff nurse in the ICU, [the issue] was that nobody wanted to send their patients to this unit because the care was so poor. After a while, [that perception] really changed and clinically it was a great unit. The satisfaction is that all these issues I had in the beginning are better. I have seen the improvement. I have fixed some of it.

They Seek Change Through New Learning

A TCAB nurse manager detailed her attraction to change through learning, and explained how it was linked to her engagement: "I love to volunteer us for new adventures. I am committed to being the best, but getting there in a fun way, to encouraging people to see new opportunities both on and off the job."

Nurse educator Kerfoot (1998) notes that managers behave like leaders when they become "continual learning machines." The data collected in the NME study provide examples of nurse managers' personal and professional development through education, projects, and new positions that involve risk taking and innovation. Like the manager from Cincinnati, their attraction to new learning serves as a model of change agility to their staff.

Examples from Interviews

I think that one of the reasons I stay and I continue to do what I do is to receive each day as a learning experience, so that every day I'm taking away new things and learning more about myself. I've had lots of experiences and opportunities to really grow and develop personally in some of the initiatives that I have been involved with. I think because I continue to grow in my own life and to be a better person and therefore be a better leader while I'm here, that makes me want to continue with what I'm doing and also help others to do the same.

I think the strength is that there are so many opportunities here to do whatever anyone would want to do in different capacities. Over the years with my time in this position, the greatest learning and growth opportunities have been being able to participate in projects or initiatives that are beyond the unit's goal and to really be involved in something bigger, something hospital-wide. Knowing that those opportunities are out there is the reason that I don't think about going somewhere else. Everything that I want is here. I can't imagine there being something better somewhere else. One of the things we notice, being in the position that we're in, [is that] when things go well or people see that we have strengths and we can do something really powerful, we'll be given other responsibilities. It's never boring. There are always new opportunities. Having had all those different experiences and opportunities, I think each one of them has helped me grow and be a better person, a better leader, and just better in general. It has stretched me in ways I never thought of.

AFFIRMATIVE FRAMEWORK

To understand the importance of a nurse manager's affirmative framework, consider its opposite. Raise your hand if you remember showing up for the night shift

- Uses an optimistic explanatory style
- Generates positive expectations
- Models resilient behavior

and being welcomed with a sarcastic greeting: "I hope you had a nap, because you have a great night ahead of you!" By contrast, engaged nurse managers might view this situation as an example of what former AONE president Marilyn Bowcutt called "a great opportunity brilliantly disguised as an impossible situation."

The importance of resilient thoughts and behaviors to prevent nursing burn-out and longevity is well established (Leigh-Edward & Gylo-Hercelinsky, 2007; Leigh-Edward & Warelow, 2005). The use of an optimistic thought process to create a positive framework for events and expectations is a cornerstone of resilient behavior (Seligman, 1992). Three aspects of the element of this frame-work drive nurse managers' capacity for engagement.

They Employ an Optimistic Explanatory Style

Here is a classic story about a manager's optimistic explanatory style: "A nurse came up to me and complained, 'there are 40 people in this person's family and they are totally blocking us. If we have to do CPR, we'd be in a predicament.' And my response was, 'How wonderful. This person has 40 people here to see them. You need to open your mind.'"

Psychologist Martin Seligman (1992) defines "explanatory style"—what you say to yourself during challenging events—as a key to resilient thinking and behavior. Kegan (1983) called this inner conversation "composing the event." The NMEP data reveal that optimistic explanatory style allows managers to interpret stress in a way that allows them to meet the challenges they face.

Examples from Interviews

> I am incredibly optimistic. What I offer is to say, "It's not that bad." You know, "Let's just take [the situation]; let's just try to objectify it; let's try to depersonalize it and pick up and go from here. What do we really want to happen? What will really help us get there? You know, all these feelings aren't really going to help. You can let some of that go and then move forward and set some new goals. Maybe they'll be smaller or [we will have] a little struggle with something." I feel like I do that all the time. And I do it with my peers also: "It's alright. You know what? Things like this happen, and it's not that out of the ordinary. Let's just take a deep breath and think about what we want to have happen and try not to dwell on the past."

> You will not see me walking down the hallway with a grumpy face and not smil-ing. I think those are the things that I hear—that you are always smiling, you have a good attitude, you have a positive attitude. I am a very positive person. Even if the worst thing could happen, I always look at the positive side. This is the worst thing that can happen; what else can we see that could happen that would be good? There is always that positive attitude from me. I have never seen the negative; it has always been that positive.

They Generate Positive Expectations

The capacity to envision and anticipate a positive outcome has been correlated with motivation, perseverance, and increased probability of goal attainment

(Bird, 2001; Scheier & Carver, 1992; Seligman, 1992). In the NMEP study, this aspect was revealed in terms of positive expectations about people and situations. Here is one manager's mantra: "We can do it. We will make it work. We want to do it. Here is how we can do it."

Examples from Interviews

> I am a firm believer that there is not a problem in the world that cannot be solved. I think my husband is going to put that as my epitaph. We need to work together and trust the people who you're on a team with. It's not that I never get stressed or that I don't have reactions, but when pressure is high, I tend to calm down. I tend to step in. Even when I was a charge nurse, I would step in to a terrible situation and say, "I need you to do this, I need you to do that, and that is all I need you to do, and we all are going to fix it." Just step in and say, "We will get through it."

> I ultimately believe in the goodness of people. I have heard other people ask me why I am surprised when I hear something [negative] that other people have said about other units. They wonder how I can still believe after all that. I really don't know but I try to look at the positive part and not totally get mired in the negativity. . . . So I do have a genuine liking for people, even people who I really don't know but I've heard [about] and was a little fearful in dealing with. I can tap into something . . . that is positive at least and maybe not make them as angry.

> I treat people like they had the best of intentions, [even] if they didn't. Actually, I just think that way. That's just how I think—but I do it intentionally, too. If somebody [does] something and it seems counterproductive to the team, I see it as "You were trying to help that patient, weren't you?" And I'll give them a way to say it [so] they can show that they had good intentions. Whether or not it was true, sometimes [the point is] to get them to think that it was true.

They Model Resilient Behavior for Staff

The NMEP interviews indicate that use of a resilient framework is not only part of an individual manager's behavior, but also a deliberate action that provides a model for staff to emulate. Said one nurse manager, "I don't let the stress show to the staff. I think they take that from me. I'll tell them, 'This is okay. We have seen this before, and we are going to get through this.'"

Examples from Interviews

> I thought my hair would go on fire yesterday. That was yesterday, and today is a new day. I think all of those things. I think it's also what you make it. You can come here and be the most miserable person. Life is too short. I do my share of complaining, I admit it. But you know, you have to get over that and move on, because if you

stay with the negativity and complaining, then your hair will always be exploding. It's not worth it. If you walk around like that, then your staff turns into that [image]. If they see your hair is on fire, then their hair is on fire.

I don't feel the panic. Yes, there is stress to this job and I acknowledge that, but I don't let it overcome me. . . . I think that is part of leadership. You have to set the example. If a call-off puts you over the edge, then your staff will be over the edge. That won't do anybody any good. It doesn't do any good to complain. If there is a problem, fix it.

It is instructive to compare these wonderfully detailed self-reports of the nurse managers from one-on-one interviews in the NME study with the briefer written evaluations from the chief nursing officers who selected them for inclusion in the study. Those assessments are the subject of Chapter 4.

Chief Nursing Officers on Signature Behaviors

Many of the participating chief nursing officers (CNOs) may have struggled to select only five managers with five-plus years' tenure for the Nurse Manager Engagement Study. Nevertheless, they quickly supplied the reasons why they chose the particular nurse-manager participants in the study. Five of the six CNOs also filled out a questionnaire that mirrored the appreciative inquiry approach of the NMEQ. The questions on this tool sought to discover patterns of individual signature behaviors that nurse leaders valued in their choice of participants in the study.

The CNOs answered the following five questions about individual signature behaviors for each of five nurse middle managers they selected:

1. What were the factors that made you select _____ as an outstanding nurse manager to participate in this research?
2. Let's talk about _____'s beginnings as a middle manager in this organization. What were your first positive impressions or satisfying experiences with her in the first few weeks or months? What do you think was learned or experienced during that early time that has helped her succeed over the years in the role?
3. _____ has been in the nurse manager role in your organization for at least five years. How do you explain the positive factors that have influenced her decision to stay on the job?
4. What gifts, values, attitudes, and capabilities does _____ bring to the challenges of being a nurse middle manager? How have these allowed the nurse manager to be successful, and to work long term, in this role?
5. Describe a standout or high point experience in this setting—that is, a time when you saw the nurse manager's strengths and abilities. Describe the positive factors you observed.

The results, summarized in **Figure 4–1** and **Figure 4–2**, reveal ten signature factors (listed in order of frequency of response in Figure 4–2). If these ten signature elements sound familiar, it is because seven out of the ten mirror the signature individual elements harvested from nurse manager interviews.

Signature Behavior	Behavior Specifics
1. **Affirmative Framework** "She has a positive attitude that is very calm, no matter how nutsy her unit is."	• Frames responses in resilient manner • Expresses sense of humor • Leads staff along a positive channel
2. **Change Agility** "She left the unit better than she found it."	• Leads initiatives and innovation • Thrives on challenge • Serves as a change facilitator
3. **Mission Driven** "She has a global view—she sees the implications beyond her unit."	• A vision for own unit within the larger organization • Desires to make a difference • Committed to patient population • Strong values and commitment to excellence
4. **Ardor** "She is driven and passionate. Once you meet her, you know she will be successful."	• Adores and cares for staff • Loves the people he or she works with • Displays passion for nursing
5. **Generativity** "She is growing her successor."	• Engages in succession planning • Empowers staff • Invested in the success of his or her staff
6. **Continuous Learning*** "She has used the opportunity to learn and grow."	• Loves learning • Seeks new challenges • Enriches leadership by learning from experience

Figure 4–1   Selection factors of outstanding nurse managers given by five chief nursing officers *(continues)*

Only two elements identified by CNOs—assertive communication and the capacity to command respect—did not appear as dominant themes in nurse managers' self-descriptions in their face-to-face interviews.

7. **Assertive Communication*** "She tells it like it is."	• Direct and forthright speech • Not afraid to challenge leadership • Advocates for staff and patients
8. **Attunement** "She seeks to understand rather than to be understood."	• Focuses on staff as individuals • Aware of accomplishments of staff • Listens with skill
9. **Self-Regulation** "I have not seen her in a reactive state."	• Displays steadiness and calm in high-stress situations • Quiet self-assurance
10. **Commands Respect/Confidence*** "Her sense of professional practice allows her to hold people to a higher standard."	• Mutual trust and respect • Models and demands standards of excellence

Note: Five chief nursing officers filled out the questionnaire.
*Indicates that this element was not given a prominent place in the assessments provided by nurse managers.

Figure 4–1 (continued) Selection factors of outstanding nurse managers given by five chief nursing officers

Chief Nursing Officers' Signature Selection Criteria	Nurse Managers' Self-Described Signature Behavior
1. **Affirmative Framework** Frames responses in resilient manner Expresses sense of humor Leads staff along positive channel	1. **Mission Driven** Directs orientation toward purpose and intention Focuses on end result and outcome Defines context with "big-picture thinking"
2. **Change Agility** Leads initiatives and innovation Thrives on challenge Serves as change facilitator	2. **Generativity** Finds gratification in development of others Creates a legacy Links generations Grants opportunities for autonomy and freedom
3. **Mission Driven** Has a vision for his or her own unit within the larger organization Desires to make a difference Committed to patient population Has strong values and a commitment to excellence	3. **Ardor** Conveys excitement about staff and colleagues States dedication to patient care Declares commitment to the organization
4. **Ardor** Adores and cares for staff Loves the people he or she works with Displays a passion for nursing	4. **Identification** Savors his or her part in the success of the staff Maintains a clear a line of sight to the care of the patient at the bedside Creates an atmosphere where staff can provide superb patient care
5. **Generativity** Engages in succession planning Empowers staff Invested in the success of his or her staff	5. **Boundary Clarity** Cultivates strong internal boundaries Creates emotional insulation Restores boundaries through disengagement Models and displays appropriate boundaries

Figure 4–2 Ranked comparison of CNO signature selection behaviors and nurse managers' self-described signature behaviors (continues)

6. **Continuous Learning**
Loves learning
Seeks new challenges
Enriches leadership by learning from experience

7. **Assertive Communication**
Direct and forthright speech
Not afraid to challenge leadership
Advocates for staff and patients

8. **Attunement**
Focuses on staff as individuals
Is aware of the accomplishments of staff
Listens with skill

9. **Self-Regulation**
Displays steadiness and calm in high-stress situations
Displays a quiet self-assurance

10. **Commands Respect and Confidence**
Generates mutual trust and respect
Models and demands standards of excellence

6. **Reflection**
Leverages lessons from experience
Observes the effect of his or her own behavior on others
Scans for cues about self and others in workplace

7. **Self-Regulation**
Suspends judgment before acting
Uses restraint to keep emotions in check
Practices perseverance
Cultivates patience

8. **Attunement**
Shows regard for the individual and appreciation for each person's contribution
Understands diverse perspectives
Sets aside assumptions

9. **Change Agility**
Challenges the process through innovation
Welcomes and initiates change
Seeks change through new learning

10. **Affirmative Framework**
Uses an optimistic explanatory style
Generates positive expectations
Models resilient behavior

Figure 4–2 (continued)   Ranked comparison of CNO signature selection behaviors and nurse managers' self-described signature behaviors

The data suggested some intriguing overlap. For example, when CNOs described the element of continuous learning, they included elements of reflection (learns from experience), and their descriptions of generativity included an element of identification (invests in success of her staff). Clearly, the consistency of the factors suggests the promise that might be realized by focusing on these signature elements in the process of engagement education, as discussed in the final chapter of this book. An additional powerful finding is the ordering of the data. While nurse managers rated an affirmative framework as the last ranked of ten dominant elements, the CNOs who selected this factor rated it as number one on their lists.

The alignment of the data has important implications for the recruitment, training, and continuing education of nurse managers. For example, senior leadership clearly prizes the capacity for resilient thinking and behavior, and nurse managers count it among their assets in success. This concurrence suggests two future directions in using this information. First, there is a need for identification of affirmative frameworks in managers being recruited and hired. Second, there is a demand for education and training to develop this capacity in both new and long-time managers. These applications will be discussed in Chapter 7.

Before we consider these topics, all applications must be considered in the context of what nurse managers can teach us about building cultures of engagement.

CHAPTER 5

Signatures of Organizational Culture

Creating questions to prompt nurse managers to describe their organizational culture—one where they work each day—reminded me of a story told by the novelist David Foster Wallace. An older fish asks a younger fish, "How's the water?"And the young fish answers, "What's water?"

Similarly, the challenge of asking managers to identify details of their organization's culture was like asking them to describe the water where they swim every day. Several questions in the NMEQ were carefully designed to harvest specifics about organizational values, aspirations, and support.

The responses from managers suggested both an informal sense of "the way we do things around here" and more specific elements of organizational culture in terms of shared assumptions, values, and beliefs about the accepted and expected ways of acting (Cooke & Lafferty, 1989). These comments also conveyed a sense of the ethos of the organization—the prevalent tone or spirit of the community and its habitual patterns of commitment. They call to mind the definition of ethos as the genius of an institution (Harris, 1993).

Healthcare culture is a strong focus of research and is clearly linked to nurse manager engagement (Ingersoll & Kirsch, 2000). Littell (1995) described the perception of organizational climate as the most important predictor of job satisfaction of mid-level nurse managers. Kane-Urrabazo (2006) found that strong organizational culture predicted middle manager strategic involvement.

Engaged nurse managers described five signature organizational factors that contributed to their longevity and their engagement:

- Learning culture
- Culture of regard
- Generative culture
- Culture of meaning
- Culture of excellence

Since the NMEP study's completion, these factors have continued to be illuminated in classes and dialogues with hundreds of nurse managers.

LEARNING CULTURE

A nurse manager defined learning culture with great enthusiasm: "It's a great learning experience and they always provide training for you. There are always options for you—continuing education, advancement of jobs if you want to." Notably, managers from all six medical centers in the NMEP seconded her emotion.

- **Create opportunities for educational mobility**
- **Encourage learning through risk taking and increased visibility**
- **Provide transparency and accessibility of information and resources**

The phrases "learning organization" and "learning culture" have been used to describe an organization that builds a community of learners, and that invests in individual learning to enhance the organization as a whole (Chan, 2001; Senge, 1990; West, 1994). And there is more: sustained employee engagement has been linked to an organizational support of learning and growth (Wagner & Harter, 2006) as well as providing the information and resources necessary to accomplish work (Kanter, 1993; Laschinger, 2005).

In designating their organization as a learning culture, managers in the study and the classroom illustrated three aspects of this signature element.

Create Opportunities for Educational Mobility and Continuous Learning

A long-time manager from Oahu described a leadership class in her organization and noted its potential for continuous learning: "all of the managers come together to learn, discuss, and share. Even for those of us who have worked together for years, it is during these classes that facades come down."

Two salient characteristics of learning organizations are continuous learning opportunities (Clavert, 1994; Watkins & Marsick, 1993) and educational mobility (Melnyk, 2006) through accessible advanced education. Managers emphasized the availability of ongoing education and opportunities for advanced training and degree completion.

Examples from Interviews

In the management role, they have given me the tools that I need. They focus on education, whether it be formally or informally. We have a wonderful administration that finds value and puts their money where their mouth is as far as providing educational support to me as well as to staff members, such as the advanced practice nurses, providing conferences and sending people to conferences.

I have had great opportunities to do things [that I] never in my wildest dreams knew I would be doing. They had me participate in some focus groups; I presented a couple of posters—I've never done that prior to coming here. I didn't think the things I did were worthy of those [recognitions] when, in fact, they were really quite cool. I came here with a master's in healthcare administration. So I have a degree in teaching, a BSN, a master's in healthcare administration, and I have another two classes and I will finish my MBA.

In the last ten years I have traveled as far as Finland to go to an international nurses symposium. Two weeks ago [I was] in Boston; this fall I'm going to Denver and Miami. It's amazing. I was in San Diego a few years back and I never thought in nursing you would travel if you weren't a traveling nurse, and yet I am getting this opportunity to learn [with] the best in the country and to be a part of it.

They gave us enough education; they provided us with advanced leadership classes. They provided us with classes here and they sent us to seminars outside to enhance our specialty. So education is good here—we have the master's program [right here] for MSN.

Encourage Learning Through Risk Taking and Increased Visibility

This aspect of a learning culture is captured in the words of a TCAB nurse manager from Chicago, who recalled how her chief nursing officer had encouraged her to make a presentation at a national meeting: "I respected her and knew that she valued and trusted me to accomplish this. I enjoyed it, and learned that I could be a public speaker, and was a success after all."

Learning healthcare organizations are also defined by opportunities to practice new skills and competencies, and by their creation of a climate that facilitates and rewards learning (De Burca, 2000). Challenging assignments have also been identified as a critical factor for leadership development (CCL, 1990).

An AONE nurse manager fellow gave this example:

I had only been in my role for two months when my senior director assigned two of us to make a presentation to the joint replacement center's leadership. [She] probably knew all the answers, but she asked us what we wanted to present for each part and allowed us to be present. The outcome was that the project was completed [and] well received, and that two new directors learned a lot about presenting and mentoring.

Nurse managers spoke frequently of being encouraged to take risks to learn and to become more visible. As a manager explained, "the greatest learning and growth opportunities have been being able to participate in projects or initiatives that are beyond the unit's goal and to really have been involved in something bigger, something hospital-wide."

Examples from Interviews

> Right now I am involved in implementing [a new project]. That's a pretty lofty task and I'm stumbling with it at certain points, but I still have never felt anybody not have confidence in me to be able to follow it through. It has really pushed me to [make presentations] at conferences related to falls. This is totally out of my comfort zone, but [the organization has] supported me 100% financially.
>
> Our administrator is very good at exposing, at getting others in the organization to see and notice us. She makes sure that we present, at patient operation meetings, where all the nursing leadership is. She'll put you out of that comfort level and push you out there slowly to say, "Okay, get recognized. Make sure that we're on hospital-like committees." When she's not present, we're there representing her.
>
> Knowing that those opportunities are out there is the reason that I don't think about going somewhere else. Everything that I want is here. One of the things we notice, being in the position that we're in, [is that] when things go well or people see that we have strengths and we can do something really powerful, we'll be given other responsibilities. It's never boring. There are always new opportunities.

Provide Transparency and Accessibility of Information and Resources

Knowledge accessibility has been defined in terms of the availability and clarity of job-related information and resources (Bassi & McMurrer, 2007). Managers detailed accessibility in terms of the importance of "go to" people, transparent organizational structure, an in-depth formal orientation, written manuals, and resources. Transparency was also linked to availability: "anytime I had a question, I could pick up the phone."

Examples from Interviews

> I also know who my resources are, and I can rely on other people whether they are other managers [or not]. I have become friends with some colleagues. You know who you can bounce things off of. Other departments [are also] resources—for example, human resources, knowing who your person is and who the director is. You know that you do have backup and if you have questions, there is somebody there.
>
> Being a new manager, I knew I had a lot of things to learn with the system—knowing the other nurse managers and the other managers of the other service lines. I had resources—it was very easy to find someone. I went through a new

manager's orientation. We had these huge binders and handouts [that said] if you needed somebody, this is where you were going to call. It was very easy to pick up the phone and call somebody, and they were very willing to direct you to the right person. It seemed like the first two weeks [the organization] was huge and too many people, but I was able to find my way easily.

I still have my manual, and I still refer to it. At the end of the day you are fully saturated with information, but you take this handbook with you. When the time comes, you really need that; . . . I can go back and [the manual lists] step-by-step things to do with payroll, our time and attendance, if you have problems with that, and this is the toll-free number you have to call. It is very, very good.

It was very important to know the key people and the key resources . . . you could not think enough if you had problems with employees, . . . those are the number one personnel issues that take a lot of your time. But if you know who to call and who you are directed to, you call your HR specialist. If someone has been sick, you call the employee health services. That is the information that I took with me up to this time, and it was very helpful. If we didn't have that, I would be lost in the dark and it would be hard for me to just spend my time searching.

There were certain unit directors who were good at certain things. If I didn't know how to do something with the scheduling system that we had, there was a certain individual I could call for that. If it was a payroll question, it was a different person. We just focused on who had the strength in what areas. One person wasn't your contact. I learned the "go to" people from the unit director who was on the sister oncology unit. She knew who to call, and if she did not know the answer, she would refer me to that person. I was given a list of who does this well. It was like, "I don't know how to help that. Why don't you call this person?" . . . when you realized which unit directors had the strengths in which areas, it seemed to help.

CULTURE OF REGARD

In a conversation about cultures of regard, a long-time nurse manager from Indiana described her organization's response to what had been called "the 500-year flood" that devastated the entire hospital and closed down all of its operations for several months: "During the shutdown, our CEO insisted upon keeping all 1800

- **Convey esteem for nursing through responsiveness to viewpoint, and decision making of managers**
- **Empower nursing practice; facilitate goal attainment**
- **Foster collegial physician–nurse relationships and accountability**
- **Make small gestures of support**

employees on the regular payroll. This is a testimony to valuing employees. I have never heard of this happening in other places."

The descriptor "culture of regard" is derived from Robert Kegan's (2002) discussions of the language of regard and the value of being valued. Nurse managers in the NMEP study and in the classroom spoke of their organizations' ability to convey regard as a foundation of their engagement.

Research that maps positive organizational support (Eisenberger, 1986; Laschinger & Purd, 2007) has suggested that employees form beliefs about how much organizations value their contribution and care about their well-being. These beliefs about being well regarded by organizations have been linked to positive emotional commitment to the organization (Rhoades & Eisenberger, 2001) and described as drivers of engagement (Robinson & Perryman, 2004) and high levels of performance (Patrick & Spence-Laschinger, 2006).

A TCAB nurse manager, when asked for an example of organizational support, recalled a problem her unit was having with a subspecialty team at a meeting: "our CNO came and supported us, and our concerns. I think it is very hard for nurses to speak out against practice of physicians, and she role-modeled how to have a difficult conversation." Another manager said simply, "I never felt out on a limb."

Creating a culture of regard connects the dots between the nurse manager's engagement and the engagement of staff nurses. Intriguing research suggests that supervisors who feel supported by their organization reciprocate this support with their staff (Shanock & Eisenberger, 2006). Regard for managers is something that is played forward. Data collected via the NMEP study interviews identified four interrelated elements in cultures of regard, which have been emphasized in classes and conversations since the study's completion.

Convey Esteem and Recognition of the Significance of Nursing

The construct of organization-based self-esteem (OBS) has been defined as the extent to which employees perceive themselves as important, meaningful, and effective within their organization (Gardner, 1998; Pierce & Gardner, 1989). Nurse managers interviewed for the NMEP study and those participating in subsequent classes I have taught gave general and specific examples of the high esteem assigned to, and positive valuation of, nursing in their organizations. The value was also stated in relation to medical staff. A manager summed this factor up by saying, "From the organization, there is an acknowledgment and understanding of the work [of nursing]; there is respect."

Examples from Interviews

Nursing is a voice—not to the exclusion of anybody else, but they are definitely a player at the table, so to speak. I always felt issues that had to do with patient care would be addressed on the same level as any other department. That has always made me feel that it is very important to be here to be part of that . . . that is probably why I would be less likely to move somewhere else. Nursing per se is very important to me, and if that is not going to be an integral part of the organization, then I don't really want to be a part of that.

Nursing here is very strong. It is intentional, and that is a huge thing to me. Our medical staff is very supportive of nursing. The older residents will say, "what's going to make or break it here for you is the nurses, so be careful that you listen to them."

We had a situation about 18 months ago, [involving] one of the newer doctors who had been here as a fellow and everyone really liked him. After he became an attending [physician], he kind of got a big head and was acting kind of weird, and we didn't know what was going on. The medical director told him he had to come to resolve [the issue] with me. If he was going to continue to work here, he had to resolve it with me. He came in to meet with me and we talked. . . . I told him the nurses didn't feel that he respected them anymore.

   I told him that I knew that I was much older than him and I was not at the bedside, but I wanted him to know what was going on. I know there are hundreds of nurses here and just one of him, and I told him he had to have a relationship with them and treat them respectfully or he would sink. I told him we needed to figure out what he had to change. I would tell the nurses to step up, but he would need to meet them halfway. He was really shaky about it, but he went out and did what I asked him to do. About a week later, people started saying he had really changed. He told me later that it was working. That would not have happened if the medical director had not talked to him about rectifying this [problematic situation].

Empower Nursing Practice: Be Responsive to the Manager's Viewpoint and Decision Making

Studies of empowerment in nursing practice have demonstrated the links between high autonomy and increased role satisfaction, high-quality care, and retention of nurses (Aiken & Patrician, 2000; Kramer & Schmalenberg, 2003). Listen to a manager in San Francisco describing this esteem: "nurses are valued as members of the interdisciplinary team. Nursing is represented at all of the important decisions."

   Empowerment was framed in terms of the organization's responsiveness to nursing managers' viewpoints and decisions. "The directors I had were not micro-managers. You have the flexibility, you have the autonomy to do what is best for your unit—and they will always stand behind you in your decisions," one manager said.

Examples from Interviews

. . . but just their openness to hear recommendations and ideas, their openness to removing barriers, just their overall support. They tour through the areas periodically. The staff may not be aware of who they are. They do it relatively unobtrusively. Then sometimes they come and everyone knows exactly who they are. It's just interesting. I think they're overall supportive, they're overall encouraging. I've never had the sense that any of them have felt like, "I don't really have time for you, for this."

The openness and encouragement to run with your ideas . . . I feel like they respect me as a person and as a professional and the ideas that I bring forth, even though they might be a little rough around the edges. I may not articulate it well; I may not use the proper terminology or whatever. They never make you feel like, "Wow, you shouldn't have done that; you shouldn't have said that."

The institution has been very, very supportive if I bring something to the table and I can demonstrate why it is important from [a standpoint of] either recruitment or attention or a patient care–related issue, regardless of the fact that it may or may not be outside the budget that we all have to live with, because this is a business. I have had support. I haven't had to jump over hurdles. [I have had] the ability to work through an organization that doesn't make me prove myself from day one.

[I used almost a priori knowledge] of how do you determine how many nurses you need and present a proposal from every layer up, building. . . . At that meeting, basically Mr._____ turned to me and the medical directors and said, "You know how to run your department, you know what you need." He handed me, verbally, a virtual blank check for 13 more FTEs [full-time equivalents].

That trust which translates into an awful lot of money, that trust in financial survival, that trust in organizational skills, that not having to ask me to show him all the paperwork and all the formulas I created to get to this, because there really weren't that many, was tremendously empowering. Right from the beginning [they said] to me, "Yes, you do know what you know, and you need to feel comfortable with it, and you need to share it with us because that's one of the reasons we brought you here. We brought you here because you can hit the ground running as a manager, and you can hit the ground running in terms of your knowledge, your clinical knowledge and expertise."

Facilitate Goal Attainment

Another facet of perceived organizational support and regard is facilitating attainment of the manager's goals. This can include creating access to information and support, or removing in-house barriers in order to obtain the desired results (Kanter, 1993; Manion, 2005). Put simply, this means, "they were there to help us get it done."

Examples from Interviews

This is the best place in town, the reason being that they really care about their employees in a manner where they want you to tell them what resources you need in order to reach the outcome, that all of us are looking for. That is how I see this place and, like I said, I have been to other hospitals. I said to the nursing staff, "you are the most spoiled rotten nurses in the whole world—not just in the United States, in the whole wide world; everything is at your fingertips."

Within nursing, the leadership is very supportive at the director level; the directors are supportive of one another. The organization seeks director input in decision making and problem solving, which then demonstrates support and respect. If something negative happens, there is support for that individual or situation. We had a family who was having a negative experience here, and they went to our CEO and chief nurse executive. They investigated what happened and how it could have been handled differently instead of just asking, "Why couldn't you create a positive experience for this family?" They handled it in a supportive way instead of a negative accusatory way.

I think they are very, very supportive of the middle manager role. They have done so many things. We have monthly meetings with no administration present, just the unit directors. We had our own nominal group technique. We went through our list of what we needed to do to succeed. They supplied us with the resources to make this happen. They have always been there with the mindset that this is our job and what do we need to get it done. They were there to help us get it done.

Make Small Gestures of Support

Managers demonstrated strong awareness of small gestures of positive organizational support (Eisenberger, 1986; Laschinger & Purd, 2007; Patrick & Spence-Laschinger, 2006; Rhoades & Eisenberger, 2001) and spoke about how these moments contributed to their beliefs that the organizations valued their work and cared about their welfare. As my mother Selma, a former nurse manager, used to say, "little things mean a lot." One AONE nurse manager fellow wrote about a director who had been working with her on salary and budgeting, "He called me at home and walked me through my weekly payroll, so I would be successful. Many times my director will walk me through meetings prior to the actual get-together, so that the outcome will be a success."

Examples from Interviews

They do a lot of different things that show support of the organization. We have a teacart that comes out to the staff for tea breaks, for staff who can't go off the unit. It has chocolates and apples and hot tea. We do something called quiet time every day at 2:00 p.m., where we shut down the lights in the hallways and dim the lights in the nurses station for that half-hour from 2:00 to 2:30, so that nurses can regroup in their day. You are supposed to try to be quiet and only talk when you need to talk for that half-hour from 2:00 to 2:30, so that nurses can regroup in their day. If you go in units, you will see the lights all dimmed low.

> We have senior nurses recognition days, for nurses [who have been here for] over five years. Of course, Nurses Week is always a big deal around here. The VP of nursing and the nurse executive group come in and do night rounds couple of times a year to meet with the night staff. So there are a lot of little things that we do. It's probably something monthly that recognizes that you are doing a good job or we're looking at your role as a nurse, whether it's "let's give them 12-hour shifts" or "let's do a weekend program"—we are always looking out for what we can do to recruit and retain our most valued resource, our nurses.

CULTURE OF MEANING

Organizations with clear cultural values and priorities—those that define the essence of meaningful work—were drivers of engagement in the study data as well as in educational sessions and

> • **Communicate with clarity about the organization's mission and values**
> • **Foster alignment of individuals' and the organization's goals and values**

meetings with nurse managers since the study's completion. A recent example illustrates this point. When asked about how her organization had been a good fit in enhancing her success and longevity, a manager of several decades answered, "It is a culture that is relationship-based—at my peer level and at the staff level. Administrative changes have made that more difficult, as more 'for profit' cultures are entering. But, so far, this hospital is still far more relationship based."

Studies of nursing environments have defined meaningful work in terms of individuals being clear about the organizational mission, sharing the organization's values and goals, and finding satisfaction in their own contributions to those goals (McManus & Monsalve, 2003). Personal engagement has been linked to employees creating meaningfulness on the job (Kahn, 1990; Wagner & Harter, 2006).

The NMEP data revealed four out of the six organizations to be cultures of meaning as demonstrated in two related ways. Both aspects link cultures of meaning to the individual signature of being mission driven.

Provide Clarity About Mission

The importance of clarity and perception of mission in nursing environments has been described by McManis and Monsalve (2003). The management of meaning has been described as a key element of leadership (Bennis, 1989).

In the study data, nurse managers' descriptions detailed their mindfulness about the institutional values and goals: "Our hospital vision is to create a brighter future for all children. It is very simple—but complicated." Notably, this organizational element is aligned with the individual signature behavior of being mission-driven.

Examples from Interviews

> In everything that I have tried to do or have done, the question is always, "Is it the best thing for children and their families?" That was always the question. I remember that as a new grad and even as of yesterday. That reinforces to me that it is truly the mission. No matter who is in the president's role or any role, that if they ask that question there is some sense that they believe it, too.
>
> I think the factor that really, really keeps me in one place, it has to be [this hospital's] balance and philosophy. I always refer back to that. We look at service for the poor, and I'm looking further than that, looking at foreign countries, poorer countries, [where] the kids have diseases, and they just don't have resources to help them and to give them service. The philosophy here has taught me to see the wider scope and to look at things around me. I don't just look at a patient's financial problem and they come to us, to this hospital to treat them, but I look further than that.
>
> Our nursing officer has a vision and a value of [the importance of] and a desire to have it continually stretch and grow and be professional. She values the bedside nurse as much as the advanced practice nurse and as much as the nurse manager. All of us make up the matrix of what nursing is. Her vision for that, her pushing you to do better, her saying she will meet us halfway, her ability to set a standard and a position nationally give us that external pride. The whole world is watching [this hospital.] I want to do better and I want to make her proud of me because that is reciprocal in how proud I am of her representing where I work.

Foster Alignment Between Organizational and Individual Values

Engagement has been linked to the alignment and fit of what is important to an organization and its members (Spence-Laschinger & Finegan, 2005). Alignment contributes to a personal connection to the mission and meaning of working in an organization (Gallup, 2006). Kahn (1990) calls this a return on investments of self. As one manager put it, "This institution emphasizes relationships, and that seems to be my personal belief also." Another respondent named this alignment as a touchstone: "The factor that really, really keeps me in one place, it has to be this hospital's balance and philosophy and service to the poor. I always refer back to that."

Examples from Interviews

> The majority of people here are aligned with the mission. I actually see very few people who aren't, and if they aren't, they're either assisted in aligning themselves with the mission or it just ultimately isn't a good fit for them within the organization. It seems to me—and I'm not sure why exactly this is—but I really see that

> [this place] draws people in who tend to have more of that collegial relationship, more of that teamwork, that sense of community. And maybe it is because of the mission; maybe the majority of the people hire on because they feel some sense of relation or obligation or respect for the mission.

> This gives me the feeling of pride. This institution has emphasized these relationships, and that seems to be my personal belief also. It's the emphasis on quality and patient care, not the bottom line, even though that is obviously the role we live.

GENERATIVE CULTURE

A nurse manager from Virginia described her organization's vice president of nursing as "someone who helps me to succeed every day by developing me professionally. We entered a [TCAB] storyboard competition and

- **Provide guides and exemplars to mentor the next generation**
- **Provide visible role models**
- **Offer available and approachable leadership**

won first prize. It was a high point of my career." Contrast this statement with the words of a brand-new nurse manager: "My unit is the only reason I stay. I am not receiving mentorship, despite repeated requests. This gives[me] a sense that nurse managers are replaceable."

These examples illustrate key points from the emergent study of organizational generativity (Cooperrider, 2007), which includes documenting the organizational activities that are "generative" in character (i.e., actions that take care of the next generation). The signature elements of generative nursing cultures, like those of generative individuals, are defined by a multifactor commitment to caring for, and contributing to, the next generations (Erikson, 1950; McAdams, Hart, & Maruna, 1998).

Nurse managers from four of the six medical centers in the NMEP suggested generative culture as a dominant element that was reflected in three specific ways. In addition, when they listed wishes for future nurse managers (see Chapter 6), they underscored the importance of a mentor or preceptor as a dominant theme.

Provide Visible Mentorship

Mentoring relationships have been linked to nurse manager engagement (Grindel, 2003), career goal attainment, and talent management (Spengel & Parsons, 1997; Wilson, 2005). In the NMEP data, the description of mentorship went beyond teaching, training, and sharing skills relationships. Many managers echoed the comment, "She taught me everything I could know about nursing."

Managers in many settings talked about mentors as being the ones who socialized them to the role, values, customs, and resources of the profession (Pataliah, 2002) and offered opportunities for reflection and learning about nursing practice (Grindel, 2003). The vast majority of the managers in the NMEP study talked about having a significant mentor or guide. These descriptions offered a front-row seat to observe themes and variations of cultures that are characterized by generativity.

Examples from Interviews

There are a probably a few examples that I could give for that. I succeeded, and they have pushed me along. They backed me all the way.

One standout is [name]. She was my boss, and she really helped me when I started up the unit. She helped me with the transition and to become acclimated. I had a whole new peer group. I went from being a nurse manager on the surgical floor to being a nurse manager on a medical floor, so there were a different group of nurse managers who were my colleagues and my peers. I would say she helped me succeed in that area. She was supportive. She helped me with staffing, and I pretty much got whatever I asked for. She helped me to get an assistant nurse manager and as far as staffing, whatever I needed, she backed me on. She taught me a lot about the way the service runs and what her expectations were. She was very supportive . . . during that first initial year that I was making that transition.

A mentor [is] somebody who I can trust, someone who I can go to at any time. Last week . . . multiple things went down. I can go to her and vent for five minutes and get those frustrations out because if I don't, I'm going to blow up on the unit. I know I can call her and vent and, in five minutes, I'll feel much better. I can then be a better manager. [It's great] just having someone that you can do that with. I don't feel I can do that within my peer group. I can do that with my clinical director. I don't think she looks at it as not being a good manager but having reached a [certain] point, and she knows when I have reached my point. I feel supported in that way, because I think we all need that person who we can go to, when you get to that point, just needing five minutes to vent. Then you can relook at the situation. She will reel me back in. She says, "Why don't you go do this now?" This is supportive in my mind. . . . I think we all need to have that person who we can go to, who we trust enough to say, "I'm having a bad day." Believe me, she puts me in line or she will tell me when I'm not doing something right. She'll tell me when I'm wrong and will lead me.

He would say, 'Talk to me. I know you are thinking. What are you thinking? Let me hear you." I never had somebody like this in my career. I didn't have any director or somebody [to whom] I reported that his title was also very different, so I think he was my mentor. He would keep asking me a lot of questions that I never even thought about, so it made me think. "Why do you really need this neuropsychologist to be your therapist supervisor?" Sometimes I would even run

> out of answers. He would say, "You have to think about it; you need to give me a good answer." I did not go to him and ask him. He would not give me answers; he would let me think and come up with answers and then he would say, "That is what I want—now you are thinking."

Provide Visible Role Models

The importance of nurturing nurse leaders through exemplars—role models for the individual to emulate—has been described by Pataliah (2002) and Wilson and Leners (2005). Managers frequently described this sense of inspiration by example: "When I was still a supervisor, she became a director of nursing resources. I admired her knowledge and her confidence and her way of handling situations. [If I had a situation to get through,] I would ask myself, 'What would Madeleine do?'"

Examples from Interviews

> She was a very down-to-earth supervisor when I was first hired at the hospital. Yes, that was my first job. She taught me everything I could know about nursing. The way she performed things, even though [this was] way back 20 years ago. She would say, "This is how you make people feel better: Y, you do peri-care before they go to bed." She went in and did the peri-care and she was the supervisor. I learned that instead of getting a sedative to the patient, maybe we can do a little bit of peri-care to make them feel better and they go to bed. She was great: She jumped in to help, she rolled up her sleeves, and nothing was a small task for her. She taught me small things make a difference. I worked with her five years before she moved away.

> I had a very good relationship with my manager. Even way before I even considered taking the job, I think I had such a good role model that when she asked me to take the job from her, it wasn't intimidating and I didn't feel overwhelmed. I really felt that working so close with her for those first few years I was here helped me understand a lot of what was going on. [I had] positive experiences when I first started. She made it easier—she stayed around for quite a while. She kind of helped me with the parts that I didn't understand as far as budgetary parts. I knew all the clinical parts of it and the parts that involved day-to-day operations with the staff and figuring out staffing—just kind of mixing people up to make sure we didn't have holes. All that kind of stuff was easy for me because of her.

Offer Present and Approachable Leadership

The NMEP data support the work of Parsons and Stonestreet (2003), who named availability of a boss to listen and provide guidance as one of the key factors associated with nurse retention. As a manager elaborated, "I just never feel that, as bad and crazy as it may get, there isn't somebody I can go to for help to find some kind of resolution to the problem. I think that is one of the primary reasons that I stay." This kind of support creates a trickle-down economy, suggests Pinkerton (2003), who identified access to administrative support as a key factor in providing support to nurse managers and as a means of improving staff nurse retention.

Examples from Interviews

I feel supported every day. It's one of those things, when something comes up—not that it happens that often—I know that I can call my clinical director. I can call the vice president. You can go to their office if they are there. You can go to anyone's office or call him or her, and the support is there all of the time. I can't [point to] any one time, [because] it is always there. I can't recall a time when it wasn't there. It's not *hoping* that you will get the support; it's *knowing* that you will get it.

I think they are very approachable. I can call [her] and say, "I have a problem," and I will be in her office that day to go over it with her. She is hands-on. She comes to our cluster meetings in the morning. It's the hands-on [part] that makes a difference and the feeling of family and that we are friends. We have gotten bigger, but we have never lost that feeling. They are there, too, when we are starting something new and it might be a test for the staff. They are making rounds at 2:00 or 3:00 in the morning and talking to the staff, just wanting to know how things are going, how the staff feels, if there are any suggestions on how to do it better. They are right out there in the front line.

I could call them if I have a problem and it's not one of those things that [sometimes occurs when] you are in a big corporation as [this] is—that if I call or e-mail somebody I might not hear from them in 24 hours. You know that you are going to get a response, and it's going to be that same day—and a lot of times within an hour if they are not in meetings. They will assist or guide you and say, "I think you should contact this person or do this" or something that is above what you are used to dealing with on a day-to-day basis.

CULTURE OF EXCELLENCE

A TCAB nurse manager from the Midwest described her own engagement in the culture of excellence within her organization. "I feel trust and pride in knowing that we all strive to be the best in the country in what we do. This is not for bragging, but because our patients deserve it," she said.

- **Communicate high standards and expectations of excellence**
- **Cultivate brand pride and identification with the organization's accomplishments**

The idea of organizations driven by excellence was popularized by management consultants Peters and Austin (1985), and subsequently defined in nursing practice through studies of Magnet hospitals (Kramer & Schmalenberg, 1988), nursing quality management (Kruger & Wilson, 1990), and cultural excellence (Stewart-Amidei, 2003). The NMEP interview data highlighted two key facets of cultures of excellence.

Communicate High Standards and Expectations of Excellence

Knowledge of organizational expectations has been identified as one of the key factors in defining a strong organizational culture (Cooke & Roseau, 1988; Reynolds, 1986) and creating engagement (Wellins, 2007). The communication of high standards as expectations was a dominant element noted by managers in four of the six NMEP study settings. A memorable sample: "We joke about it, but it is true: 98% is never good enough."

Examples from Interviews

I have never seen this quality of care, compassion of people, dedication to always learning, and to collaborating with others. I have never seen that every day. Not just when we have a good day—we get that every day. I think that's the culture here; that's the expectation. We just maintain it.

Mediocrity is just not acceptable, and it never will be. [It is] expected [for] all of us—whether you're the janitor or you're the CEO—that you will treat people well, that you will be as helpful as you can be to them. We're going to extend ourselves to whatever degree we need to serve our children and their families.

It really is about a whole bunch of humans trying to be really good at something. That is incredibly satisfying—to be part of [a group of people who are] really trying to be good at something. Very few people in this building are here to just get stuck and stay. That's not what we are about. We are about being better and having high standards and striving.

Well, you go over the top for everything. We go to the extreme for everything. There is no "Maybe" or "Is it okay?" It has to be okay. That's not like a precedent or anything, but you just know that when you do things, they need to be done right. Like HIPAA, for instance: We are just so over the top with that. I have had surgeries elsewhere and nobody goes to the extreme that we do. The bar is high here for everything.

Cultivate Brand Pride and Identification in the Organization's Accomplishments and Reputation

Recently, a nurse manager from Kansas City spoke of her satisfaction in "knowing that our patients are getting extraordinary care." Sullivan, Bretschnieder, and McCausland (2003) describe this pride of nurse managers about their "institutional reputation." Walker (2006) refers to this kind of meaningful pride as "branding," which can become a shorthand form of identity. I have met so many nurses who spoke with pride and identification about the clinical expertise, teaching, research, and talent of their organizations. "When I go out into the community, there is no comparable nursing care to us and that makes me very proud," a manager said.

Examples from Interviews

Certainly it's [our] reputation—you know, the fact that we are doing things that are considered to be cutting edge. You know, we started doing minimally invasive open-heart surgery long before anyone else was doing it. . . . If there's something that's new out there in terms of the literature, you're going to see it [here].

I definitely take satisfaction in that—even just knowing that our survival rates for our patients are different and better than other places. I'm part of that, too—being able to be part of something that does the best that can be for patients while continually not resting on it but actively going ahead. We don't want to just believe that's self-sustaining; it takes active intentional work to sustain it and actually [become] better.

The kinds of patients who are referred to us are a plus. They often have been worked on elsewhere and have no answers, and that is challenging. [We work] with attending physicians who are going to be exposed to the teaching lesson. [We] focus on the new therapies and new technologies. We offer something that nobody else does. It just attracts such wonderful minds.

CULTURES OF ENGAGEMENT: INFORMATION AND APPRECIATION

The review of these five cultural factors—so consistently mentioned in conversations and research interviews with engaged nurse managers—makes it clear how an appreciative interview does what an exit interview cannot. By asking nurse managers unconditionally positive questions about how their organizations contribute to their engagement, we uncover data that allow organizations to learn what they are doing right. **Figure 5–1** summarizes the lessons learned.

These questions also allow managers to put their loyalty to their organizations into words. In many cases, nurse managers voiced an eloquent gratitude. Said one, "You just cannot believe what [this hospital] has given to me. It has nurtured me to grow. What I have given is very minimal compared to what has been given to me."

Still, as the next chapter suggests, while nurse managers are grateful for the strengths of their organizations, they also have a well-stated wish list.

Learning Culture
"The greatest learning and growth opportunities have been being able to participate in projects or initiatives that are beyond the unit's goal and to really be involved in something bigger."

- Creates opportunities for educational mobility
- Encourages learning through risk taking and increased visibility
- Provides transparency of information and resources

*Linked to individual signature of change agility

Culture of Regard
"He turned to me and the medical directors and said, 'You know how to run your department, and you know what you need.' He handed me, verbally, a virtual blank check for 13 more full-time employees."

- Conveys esteem for nursing through responsiveness to the viewpoint and decision making of managers
- Fosters collegial physician–nurse relationships and accountability
- Empowers nursing practice; facilitates goal attainment
- Makes small gestures of support

*Linked to individual signature of attunement

Culture of Meaning
"In everything that I have tried to do or have done, the question is always, 'Is it the best thing for children and their families?' No matter who is in the president's role, if they ask that question, there is some sense that they believe it, too."

- Communicates with clarity about the organization's mission and values
- Fosters alignment of individuals' and the organization's goals and values

*Linked to signatures of mission driven/identification

Culture of Generativity
"Her goal was to make sure that everybody was competent enough to work without her, and that is my goal. If I'm in a car accident tomorrow, they need to survive; the patients need to do well. For me, if I don't do that, I am sending them out to fail."

- Encourages visible mentors or designated preceptors
- Provides exemplars to serve as role models
- Offers available and approachable senior leadership

*Linked to individual signature of generativity

Culture of Excellence
"We joke about it, but 98% is not good enough."

- Communicates high standards and expectations of excellence
- Cultivates brand pride in the organization's accomplishments and reputation

*Four of the five signature cultural elements were aligned with individual signature elements.

Figure 5–1   The five signature elements of organizational culture

CHAPTER 6

What Do Nurse Managers Really Want?

A robust dividend of using an appreciative inquiry-based interview protocol is that it is designed as a complaint-free instrument. The questions are not intended to elicit complaints, kvetching, or blaming. This kind of inquiry empties the pockets of the usual deficit-finding question, "What's wrong here?" The opportunity for negative ruminations and fingerpointing is replaced by two positive queries: "What's working?" and "What do you want more of?"

The importance of learning the aspirations of nurse managers has been noted by Parsons and Cornett (2006). In addition to discovering signature individual and organizational factors linked to engagement, the interview protocol sought managers' perspectives on how to foster engagement of nurse managers in the future.

All participants in the NMEP study were asked two future-oriented questions based on the appreciative inquiry model of using provocative questions (Cooperrider, 1990; Whitney, 2003). The first question was designed to elicit their suggestions and aspirations for new nurse managers; the second question addressed elements they believed would bring about a desired future for the role of nurse manager.

1. If you could be granted three wishes for new middle managers coming into the field, what would you wish them?
2. Imagine this: As you drive home from work today, you slip through a wrinkle in time. It is the year 2015. All of the vacancies for nurse managers across the country are filled, the average tenure of a nurse manager is ten years, and nurse manager satisfaction is among the highest in the nursing field. What has happened to create this change?

Analysis of the NMEP data captures constructive ideas about the factors linked to engagement of nurse managers in the present and future. It also aligns with a number of the signature elements of organizations and individuals. These elements were scored based how many of the six organizations ranked them as a dominant theme in the interviews. Six themes were prominent:

- Socialization and education upon entry to management role
- Designated mentorship
- Strong physician–nurse relationships
- Work–life balance
- Compensation based on contribution
- Reduction and division of workload

In addition to the responses gathered through the 30 one-on-one interviews conducted as part of the NMEP study, 30 TCAB nurse managers from across the country and 60 AONE nurse manager fellows answered these two questions in writing. Their answers also emphasized the six dominant themes. These two groups also highlighted two other themes that had been mentioned, albeit to a lesser degree, in the NMEP study data.

SOCIALIZATION AND EDUCATION: ROLE ENTRY AND DEBUT

The theme of entry into the role—the education and socialization required in moving from staff nurse to nurse manager—has been a strong focus in nursing literature, along with the consensus that the transition cannot be based solely on clinical competence or expertise (Srisic-Stoehr & Rogers, 2004). The transition into the nurse manager role was a dominant theme in the interviews in all six organizations in the NMEP study as well as in the questionnaires completed by the TCAB nurse managers and AONE nurse manager fellows. The emphasis was on expanding the time and scope of first-year orientation to focus on both nitty-gritty issues (full-time employees [FTEs] and payroll) and leadership issues (e.g., communication techniques and interpersonal skills).

One AONE nurse manager fellow summed this issue up as "a proper orientation so that the nurse manager is truly armed with the necessary knowledge and tools for success." The focus on socialization and education of the new manager underlines the important element of enriching learning cultures.

Examples from Interviews

> I think orientation is so central. If you go diving in, you spend so much time trying to stay afloat. I see that happen too many times.

A strong orientation going into the role. Our organization is so complex. Just trying to figure out who is who and how to get something done—it's different than [in] a small organization. There are many more hoops to jump through. I honestly can't keep track of all that. I have to think for a minute and look at my list of who to call for what.

Have a leadership class that is not about management issues of timesheets and budgets, but cover leadership issues like delivering bad news kindly, communication, conflict resolution.

Learn before you jump into the position—orientation to provide tools [nurse managers] need before walking in the door, including payroll, schedules, and budget. Give them a toolbox (interviewing techniques, recruitment, budgetary class, binder with "go to" people).

I would wish them real experiential training where they would learn what skills they need early on. Not just a class where they listen, but where they can try it—that would be one. I also think [it would be helpful to have] a trainer for about a month and do things with them so [nurse managers] would not have to come in and try to figure out what things look like, what they mean, and what is important. For instance, our budgets don't look anything like the budgets across the hall or across town. Our meetings are different. It takes a while to figure out all these things. If someone could show it to [nurse managers], they would not be stumbling so. This can also include some personnel issues. For instance, what do you do if a patient gets in an argument with staff? What do you do when someone yells at you? What do you do when a staff nurse walks in and quits?

DESIGNATED MENTORSHIP: SHORT AND LONG TERM

The importance of a mentor in ensuring nurse satisfaction is well documented (Grindel, 2003; Wilson, 2005). Kan-Urrabazo (2006) found mentorship to be critical to building positive organizational culture. In the NMEP study, the need for a designated mentor in becoming a nurse manager was a dominant theme in the interviews conducted in all six organizations.

Designation of a mentor was also a key theme among TCAB nurse managers and AONE nurse manager fellows. One manager's three wishes: "A mentor, a mentor, a mentor!" One of her colleagues imagined the year 2015 as a time "when nurses mentor new nurses—rather than eating their young" and when nurse managers have "someone to help them succeed and realize that a learning curve is natural and acceptable."

These responses reflect the signature elements of generativity in both individuals and organizations. A number of managers spoke of shadowing a nurse manager, orientation by a buddy system, having a preceptor for their first few months in the role, as well as ongoing relationships. The key element was the deliberate assignment of mentors—not leaving it to chance or chemistry.

Examples from Interviews

If they are new, they should have a mentor—somebody who's right there; like you need something and you go to them and you can talk to them. It's a designated mentor. I can't imagine somebody finding a mentor on their own. I think the rest of the managers should all be mentors to a new person, so if there is one main person but so-and-so is really good at explaining the budget and so-and-so is really good at figuring out conflict and personnel issues and this and that, everybody should have an open-door policy. And they should stay tight with that person.

Start off slow with a designated mentor—someone [for] advice, contacts, direction, and emotional support. Provide a mentor to offer support during the first six months and help [nurse managers] navigate through the unwritten rules—possibly someone with institutional memory.

Having the educational support as a new manager and having another manager or director who will take them under their wing. We have some wonderful managers here. Having that peer or mentor would make a big difference in solving the little day-to-day occurrences, such as things with purchasing or human resources—just having someone you can go to when needed.

STRONG PHYSICIAN–NURSE RELATIONSHIPS: COLLEAGUESHIP AND ACCOUNTABILITY

One TCAB nurse manager asked for a magic wand to help new nurse managers "wish away any communication issues between physicians and nurses." This sense of collegial and respectful physician–nurse relationships has been associated with nurse job satisfaction (Kramer & Schmalenberg, 2003). It was a dominant theme in five of the six organizations that participated in the NMEP study. Various perspectives on strengthening physician–nurse relationships were detailed.

The aspect of physician accountability was a strong subtheme (e.g., physicians being held accountable for their behavior such as wait times and patient satisfaction, so nurses don't have to be enforcers of evidence-based practice). Increased nurse manager accountability and empowerment for decision making via physicians was also viewed as a desirable factor. These data underscore the vital importance of the signature aspect of regard as noted in organizational culture.

Examples from Interviews

[Future nurse leaders] would have to have equal standing with the medical team. This is not my personal thing, but I hear that a lot. I very often hear, "We'll do what the doctors say, but who is checking on what the doctors are doing?" Sometimes I get the impression that nurses baby-sit so that doctors can do their jobs right. Doctors need to do their jobs right. I know they are really busy, and it's not that they are not any good or not trying. Sometimes we have to do four or five steps to get them to do one step. If they could just do their one step, we would not have to do so many steps.

Our medical director has been very instrumental in getting us to work together. There was a time when they taught the nurse managers to teach the physicians how to have respectful communication with the nurses. They put us in the position of teaching the physicians, and it didn't go well. Things have changed. We now have working groups, [and] especially the buy-in of our medical directors, and this does not put the entire burden on nursing.

Nurses have to learn how to work with physicians. I have seen many nurses run and hide when a physician comes on the unit. They need to be direct with the physician, greet them, and let them know they are caring for their patient and if there is anything they need to know or do in reference to that patient care. You need to collaborate with the physician and the family. Just communication [is key]; also, working on projects together and giving input as needed. [Physicians] don't want to be hit with surprises just like we don't want to be hit with surprises. Just keep that communication open.

Make yourself present for morning rounds. [Physicians] don't want to know that you're behind office doors. They want to know that you're out there with the patients and just seeing your presence and knowing you have the commitment of your unit . . . I really think having that open communication is important, assessing what [physicians'] needs are, assessing changes that will happen, addressing their concerns immediately. Don't ignore them, even if they seem irrelevant or minimal. Give them the attention they desire. Working together in different settings or councils is important.

I'll give you an example: If a physician goes to the CNO or the CEO and complains about my unit, my response is—and I want the response from my top leadership to be—"The only person who can solve your problem right now is the manager of that unit." Because they can come back to me and say, "Doctor [X] complained about this, and that," and I would say, "You know, you should have sent him back to me because you cannot solve this problem. I am the only one who can solve this problem because it's at this level that we solve these problems."

WORK–LIFE BALANCE: REJUVENATION AND INCENTIVES

The critical importance of avoiding nurse burnout to build retention has been well established (Heckson & Laser, 2006). Managers in four out of the six organizations in the NMEP detailed ideas that contributed to work–life balance. Among them: flexible schedules (four days, ten hours), time off for rejuvenation, incentives to avoid burnout such as vouchers for dinner, and child care on campus. One manager joked, "Someone to do laundry, housekeeping, and put dinner on—anything that gives us more free time."

Balance was less of a theme with the TCAB nurse manager and AONE nurse manager fellow groups. That said, the most succinct statement of the need for balance came from a new nurse manager in San Diego, who defined balance as a combination of line of sight and self-renewal. He wrote:

> I believe that nurse managers need to feel a balance between relationship building, paper pushing, meeting attending—all the while maintaining a focus on patients and families. They need more feel good moments and fewer moments when they leave after an exhausting long day, feeling that they didn't do enough.

Examples from Interviews

> I wish [new managers] longevity. I think a life–work balance [is necessary] so that you can come back and still want to do this and not lose—and that's the challenge—the energy you have. I tell my staff, "Family comes first, and you need to have a life outside of here." I need you to be happy when you come in to work. I think that is a challenge for me. It's not that I'm unhappy; I think the challenge is balancing it off. If there were some magic way in doing these steps, I would follow them.

> [We need to] go home early. "Early" means you just finish your eight hours. You feel guilty going home on the time that you were hired for. [Nurses] should not feel guilty leaving after their 8 hours of work. . . . for me, an average day is 9 to 10 hours. I feel guilty if I go home early, because I see the other nurse managers leave the same time or later than me. [I wish] that they wouldn't feel guilty going home after 8 hours; just get your purse and leave.

COMPENSATION: TO REFLECT CONTRIBUTION AND DIMINISH STRESS

The NMEP interview data, along with written responses from TCAB nurse managers and AONE nurse manager fellows, soundly refuted economist Anthony Heye's (2005) "bad pay equals good nursing" argument. Increased pay for all nursing staff was a prominent theme in four of the six NMEP participant organizations. The comments were brief and seemed to link to the issue of pay to regard and recognition of the value of nursing practice or stress reduction.

Examples from Interviews

Salary needs to reflect the work we do.

Larger salary so people can live closer to work.

Pay bedside nurses more. Compensation should be in line with contribution.

Better pay for bedside nurses—so we can stop worrying about how to fill vacancies.

REDUCTION AND DIVISION OF WORKLOAD: ADDITIONAL PERSONNEL AND RESOURCES

In the NMEP study, the double workload of the clinical and administrative roles of nurse managers (Firth, 2002; Silvettin 2000) was addressed by managers in a majority of the organizations. They suggested a number of ways to reduce this workload, including the addition of co-managers, help with accreditation, business assistants, clinical instructors, and resources to cut down on paperwork.

Examples from Interviews

First, it would be a clinical instructor just for the unit. This person would be helping new people day-to-day, being a clinical expert, knowing policy and procedure, helping to write standards for the unit, assisting nurses with their care, being knowledgeable in medication interactions, disease entities, doing impromptu in-services—that kind of thing.

They would do the clinical things such as medications, policies, and clinical protocols—that type of thing. If there were a patient who has an interesting disease, then they would give an in-service to the staff on it maybe the next day or the day after the patient was admitted. They would help the nurses with medication teaching. They would also teach the patients. They would have patient contact as well. They would help with the orientation of the new nurses on the unit as well as beyond the six- or eight-week orientation.

Have the business assistant take some things off list that don't t require a nursing degree: schedules, assignments, payroll, filing, copying, et cetera. Hire someone to help with the paperwork.

> [We need] more computer resources to minimize paperwork—to do payroll, scheduling, more technical tools [and] resources—handheld pagers, bedside terminals.

> Hire a free charge nurse—someone able to round with physicians and support your staff.

R-E-S-P-E-C-T

The wish for respect for nursing and participation in decision making surfaced as strong themes in both the TCAB nurse managers and AONE nurse manager fellows groups. One future scenario offered by a manager summed up this point: "Senior leadership will truly recognize the strengths and quality of the nurse managers and respect and utilize their contributions." These wishes are elements of cultures of regard that had been mentioned in the NMEP wish list, albeit not with as much prominence.

Managers wrote about the need for genuine respect for the power and responsibilities and contribution of nursing. They often emphasized shared decision-making and shared governance to convey this regard.

Examples from TCAB Nurse Managers and AONE Nurse Manager Fellows

> My directors and the organization give me every opportunity to try something new. Some of my ideas work, some not so much. However, the fact that my organization trusts me to do the right things honestly takes my breath away sometimes.

> [Management will know] that equipment needs, like automatic BP machines, are just as important to nurses as computers are to a business.

> [By 2015,] a dramatic shift happened among hospital administrators where great nursing care was recognized and accepted to be the backbone of positive patient outcomes. The connection between good nursing care and supportive management was found. CNOs and directors from across the country were gathered at conferences where the findings were discussed. They went back to their hospitals with the message.

> I think if everyone on the staff could have a greater understanding of what a manager does, this would cause great manager satisfaction. There would not be as many unrealistic expectations. I know some of our staff members don't think management work is hard, as they do not know the entire behind-the-scenes work. I wish there were some grand way of letting everyone know and understand what a manager does. It is not easy work by any means.

One fellow captured the essence of these aspirations when she wrote: "This organization values the work of the middle managers by including them in all decisions necessary for positive outcomes. I think I will stay in this position because senior management always says, 'Hey, what do you think?'"

Among all groups, nurse managers were—as the saying goes—careful about what they wished for. In their aspirations, they offer a visionary and highly practical blueprint for present and future engagement. These aspirations underscore the need to turn the theories of engagement into actionable ideas.

CHAPTER 7

The Practice of Engagement: Actionable Ideas

Two questions drive the translation of engagement theory into practice: Are individual signatures of engagement a function of disposition or of education? Can nurse manager engagement be learned by individuals and practiced by organizations? The short answers are both and yes. The longer answer—regarding how individuals and organizations can develop engaged nurse managers—is the focus of this chapter.

Many nurse managers spoke of individual traits of temperament that seemed hardwired, particularly those linked to emotional mastery. Recall, for example, the affirmative framework of the nurse manager whose husband suggested her epitaph: "There isn't a problem that can't be solved." At the same time, managers talked about their traits of engagement as the result of a wisdom born of experience. Consider the nurse who learned to convey an affirmative outlook and explained, "If they see your hair is on fire, their hair will be on fire."

These accounts of learned engagement behavior bring to mind Malcolm Gladwell's (2008) studies of success. In *Outliers*, he linked the accomplishments of dozens of achievers—from the Beatles to Bill Gates—by suggesting a common denominator of "10,000 hours of practice." Nurse managers offered their own variation on this theme.

Here are some examples from the NMEP study:

I have learned over the years to be much more eloquent and state things. I used to sit there and people would say my expressions were all over my face. I have learned to [control] that much better. But I still put things out there, though, because I think it's important that nurses have this connotation for so long that "We can just fix everything; just keep giving us the dirt, and we'll just keep shoveling and put our boots on and go right through." Right, because you look like the complainer and that's not what it's about. So I have learned to rephrase things. You do get what you want when you get good at that, [but that ability] just took years and years doing it. And practice, a lot of practice: When you manage people, you practice a lot.

The first negative time you have somebody in the office because they didn't do something right—that is really uncomfortable and maybe you don't do it very well, and that person leaves feeling inadequate and that's not what you meant to happen. So the more you practice it and the more you talk and the more you say, [the better you get at this type of communication.] And be honest. I'll say, "This is an uncomfortable discussion we are going to have, and you may not like a lot of the things that I need to say, but it's important that they are said and these are the reasons why." We are here for our patients, and you get better at [communication] because you practice. *So I got ten years of practice.* I hope I'm better today than I was ten years ago, but I am open to that and to learning to do better.

At the same time, education for the engagement of individuals cannot be separated from education and transformation of cultures. The words of nurse managers reveal exemplary practices of organizations—ones that can be applied in other organizations. Consider one description of a culture of regard:

Our nursing leadership is the same way. You don't come to the table and say, "I have a problem with that;" you have at least three ideas on how you want to fix that problem. What's really neat is usually, more times than not, they will listen to you. The VP and the nurse executive group will listen to some of your ideas and often may adopt them or trial them; we test them and do different things. That is part of the nursing culture here—that you just don't say, "This is the problem," without coming with an idea, so that's what I mean about challenge—that your thinking is stimulated constantly.

This closing chapter introduces practical ideas for applying the evidence base and emerging model of engagement to individual nurse managers and their organizations. Job one is the focus on line of sight.

CULTIVATING AND MAINTAINING THE LINE OF SIGHT

Anna W. is a 40-year-old cardiology nurse who was promoted to management but quit after a year in the position. As she explained, "I was drowning in paperwork; I needed to get back to working with patients." Anna's story is a cautionary tale in the study of nurse manager engagement because the capacity to maintain a clear line of sight between supervisory tasks and patient care emerged as one of the two crucibles in ensuring managers' longevity, vitality, and excellence.

As noted earlier, one the most resonant motifs in the NMEP study was the importance of developing a line of sight (LOS) and the related idea that a nurse manager's engagement is a function of his or her capacity for meaning making. Cultivating a line of sight enhances a manager's ability to see his or her impact on direct patient care.

In the study data, three elements that contribute to maintaining the LOS—to understanding the relationship between management tasks and the outcomes of patient care—were ranked first (mission driven), second (generativity), and fourth (identification) out of the ten individual signature behaviors. In addition, the organization's ability to create a culture of meaning was one of the five positive themes linked to engagement.

In these ways, the engaged nurse manager's capacity to maintain the LOS between his or her management work, patient care, and organizational mission emerged as a central, and previously under-documented, aspect of long-term nurse manager engagement. The strength of the data underscores the need for actionable strategies for developing and maintaining LOS throughout the career of a nurse manager, including the transition from staff nurse to manager and the sustainment of a seasoned manager. Strategies for both new and long-time managers are outlined in this chapter.

The strategies presented here (and summarized in **Table 7–1**) emphasize both individual and cultural realities by putting LOS on the organization's agenda, introducing it into the cultural vocabulary, and incorporating it into teaching orientation, performance reviews, talent assessment, and assignment of support staff. Support for LOS can also be enhanced by creating opportunities to develop the dominant organizational components of identification, generativity, and mission primacy. Finally, LOS can be cultivated through quantifiable means such as evaluation of time spent on and off the unit and the management of span-of-control ratios to enable nurse managers to experience more staff and patient contact. These tools and methods, which can be used to assess and maintain a nurse manager's LOS to patient care, can be implemented in nursing education, recruitment, employment interviews, new nurse manager orientation, and coaching and mentoring of long-term nurse managers.

THE CURRICULUM AND PRACTICE OF EMOTIONAL MASTERY

The second crucible of nurse manager engagement is the capacity to handle the unique emotional challenges of the role. One promising application is the potential of a curriculum to enhance the signature behaviors of emotional mastery, including reflection, attunement, self-regulation, boundary clarity, and affirmative framework.

Table 7–1   Strategies for Creating a Line of Sight

- Introduce the idea of line of sight (LOS) into the organization's culture to create a shared vocabulary about aligning individual goals and the organizational mission.
- Involve nurse managers in rounding to enable contact with patients.
- Include explicit statements about the importance and challenge of maintaining the LOS in the transition from staff nurse to nurse manager in nursing education, job descriptions, interviews, and mentoring.
- Use behavioral interviewing to select and assess candidates' capacity for mission clarity, generativity, and identification in talent assessment.
- Create a teaching module for new nurse managers' orientation to describe and strategize about refocusing their LOS in their new role.
- Seek opportunities to streamline the work of unit managers to keep them on the unit and focused on the mission (i.e., elimination of unnecessary meetings, designation of meeting-free days, or putting the office on the unit).
- Encourage nurse managers to get out of their offices and manage by walking around—to talk to staff nurses and patients.
- Assess the span of control for all nurses and set a ratio that facilitates more staff and patient contact.
- Remove obstacles that block nurse managers' LOS to the results of patient care by evaluating their workload and adding additional personnel as needed (e.g., a clinical instructor or business assistant).
- Design annual LOS surveys that evaluate how nurse managers' time is being spent and that underline how nurse managers' work contributes to meeting goals of patient care and supporting the organization's goals and values.
- Assign each manager to write his or her own mission statement in light of the larger organization mission.
- Create visual reminders of success and reinforce performance that matters (e.g., through bulletin boards to showcase patient letters, unit scorecards, or staff achievement newsletters).
- Make stories of achievements and good news in patient care part of the daily routine in staff and management meetings and the subject of recognition notes from senior leadership.
- Include evaluation of positive identification, mission clarity, and generativity as part of performance reviews.
- Solicit nurse managers' high point experiences and contributions in evaluation and coaching sessions to create reminders of meaningful work.
- Cultivate identification with the organization through communication about accomplishments, grants, research, patient satisfaction scores, and completion of benchmarks.

In describing how she learned the art of reflection in a classroom, Sandra J., a long-time manager who participated in the NMEP study, offered a front-row seat from which to observe the process of learning to meet the emotional demands of being a nurse manager. While the capacity to reflect may not have been an endowment of her temperament, Sandra has learned and practiced this critical signature behavior. As she described her course:

> They used different personality tests—one of them was called DISC—to determine what type of a leader you are, [how] you function from an emotional standpoint, similar to Myers Briggs [a personality test]. I've also taken the Myers Briggs. [The DISC test was] similar to that in terms of identifying your style and analyzing the people who are closest to you, what their styles are (even if they don't take that DISC test), so that you could learn your own style better—learn that it was just another level of introspection so that you could be a situational manager, so you could recognize in yourself when you were being too lenient. You want to be able to have your assistant manager group learn by example, learn by mentoring. You want to not micro-manage them. Where do you draw the line in not micro-managing, but yet not abandon ing them? So by learning what my personality was and where I had control issues and where I needed to learn how to back off or communicate with them differently, [I improved my management skills].
>
> One of the things that course taught me: I had numerous people before that ask me, "How do you feel right before you lose control? Do your guts tense? Do you feel your hands tighten?—all these physical cues. I could never identify a physical cue that preceded a poor communication style. I just couldn't do it, and still haven't. But what I have learned to do from that course is to recognize what my communication style was when I was impassioned about something and when I was becoming irrational. . . .
>
> [Now] I have a mantra that I say to myself. [It's actually] two different mantras. One is slow down your speech and [the other is] lower your voice. It forces me to speak and think slower when I speak because my mind is processing so fast. As fast as I process, I tend to give the impression that what you have to say is not important because I've already gotten to the solution; I have already skipped over all of your input. That might not be the case, but I have to make myself slow down so that what you are seeing of me is that engagement, that active listening. I literally used the communication tool of taking notes with employees and saying to them at the end, "Let me review my notes." Those very simple communication tools of feedback that they taught years before really do work. Saying, "I have been doing this for years and know how to do it" is not the answer, but saying, "Okay, let me repeat this back. This is what I heard you say. Is this accurate?"—that message to an employee has been phenomenally well received.

Sandra's example, along with many others, indicates that signature elements of engagement can be learned and practiced. This suggests the possibility that a curriculum to develop emotional mastery might be introduced. It could be designed as an experiential lab course, with nurses bringing in case examples and participating in self-assessment, role-playing, and behavior rehearsal. The curriculum could be presented at two levels and in two class groupings, for both new and long-time managers.

I have had the opportunity to teach elements of an emotional mastery curriculum in several settings. The intentions and directions of this course are outlined next. The format could be a one- or two-day intensive workshop or an ongoing practicum.

OUTLINE FOR EMOTIONAL MASTERY CURRICULUM OR PRACTICUM

Objectives

To introduce five teachable elements of emotional mastery that are critical to nurse manager excellence and longevity:

- Reflection
- Self-regulation
- Boundary clarity
- Affirmative framework
- Change agility

Learning Activities

Readings, self-assessment surveys, role-playing, discussion, experiential exercises, and case studies.

Preparation

Prior to the first group meeting, participants will complete the following: the Nurse Manager Engagement Questionnaire (NMEQ), a personality inventory (e.g., DISC or Myers Briggs Type Indicator), and the online Values in Actions (VIA) strengths survey. Each participant will write up several case studies of current emotional challenges to bring to a class meeting.

Topic: Reflection

- Understand inner work—and how past relationships and experience (including successes and mistakes) shape current behavior as a manager
- Apply the Johari Window model (public self versus private self, blind spot) to scan for clues about the effect of one's behavior on others

- Introduce the appreciative inquiry model and the capacity to craft questions that drive solutions and self-awareness

Topic: Attunement

- Introduce varied listening models: empathic accuracy, content versus process listening
- Explore Edward De Bono's "six hat" model of thinking styles
- Investigate four Myers Briggs personality preferences to understand individual perspectives and strengths
- Utilize the practice of bracketing to hear the whole story and consider alternative points of view

Topic: Self-Regulation

- Practice Peter Senge's "Ladder of inference" to understand mental models and avoid jumping to conclusions
- Employ cognitive and behavioral techniques (e.g., thought stopping and thought substitution) to keep emotion and impulses in check
- Gain mastery of meta-cognition (thinking about thinking) to maintain equilibrium

Topic: Boundary Clarity

- Examine current and past situations with staff, physicians, patients' families, and administration that have generated boundary challenges
- Gain understanding of the behavior of boundary violators and learn how to respond to them
- Master actions and inner dialogue that promotes boundary clarity

Topic: Affirmative Framework

- Examine David Burn's model of countering automatic negative thoughts
- Practice using an optimistic explanatory style
- Utilize metaphors and analogy for expectancy and constraint-free analysis

Topic: Change Agility

- Use Musselwhite's change style indicator
- Employ tools for resilient thought and behavior
- Introduce the skills of facilitating change

Suggested Class Readings

Adams, J. (2005). *Boundary intelligence*. Hoboken: John Wiley and Sons.

Cooperrider, D. (1995). *Introduction to appreciative inquiry in organizational development* (5th ed.). New York: Prentice Hall.

De Bono, E. (2000). *Six thinking hats*. New York: Penguin.

Heifetz, R., & Linksky, M. (2002). Get on the balcony: Why leaders need to step back to get perspective. In M. Linsky & R. Heifetz, *Leadership on the line*. Cambridge, MA: Harvard University Press.

John, C., & Freshwater, D. (1986). *Transforming nursing through reflective practice*. Oxford, UK: Blackwell.

Kegan, R. (2002). *How the way we talk can change the way we work: Seven languages for transformation*. New York: John Wiley.

Leigh-Edward, K., & Warelow, P. (2005). Resilience: When coping is emotionally intelligent. *Journal of the American Psychiatric Nurses Association, 11*(2), 101–102.

Linsky, M., & Heifetz, R. (2002). *Leadership on the line*. Cambridge, MA: Harvard University Press.

Mackoff, B., & Wenet, G. (2004). *The inner work of leaders: Leadership as a habit of mind*. New York: Amacom.

Musselwhite, W. C., & Ingram, R. P. (1995). *Change style indicator*. Greensboro, NC: Discovery Learning.

Seligman, M. (1992). *Learned optimism*. New York: Pocket Books.

Senge, P. (1994). *The fifth discipline field book: Strategies and tools for building a learning organization*. London: Nicholas Brealey.

Vitello-Cicciu, J. (2002). Exploring emotional intelligence: Implications for nursing leaders. *Journal of Nursing Administration, 32*(4), 203–210.

THE TWO STEPS OF ENGAGEMENT: SOCIALIZATION AND SUSTAINMENT

Nurse managers revealed that cultivating line of sight and developing emotional mastery were linked to fostering the longevity and excellence that marks engagement. These behaviors must be deployed as a two-step strategy. The engaged nurse managers in the study and in the classroom offered an overwhelming consensus in linking engagement of a nurse manager to what Srsic-Stoehr and Rogers (2004) call "the debut"—the transition and socialization into the new role. This socialization must be considered as the first step in long-term sustainment of a nurse manager over time.

The following strategies can contribute to the socialization of the new nurse manager:

- Offer task assignments prior to assuming the role (to build confidence and interest in leadership as an opportunity to make an impact).
- Shadow a seasoned nurse manager as a way of understanding the demands of the role.
- Designate a mentor/preceptor from day one.

- Capture collected wisdom in a book of knowledge containing task blue-prints and a list of go to people.
- Design a formal and substantive orientation program.
- Develop a curriculum that includes administrative tasks (timesheets and budgets) as well as management and leadership skill enhancement (both interpersonal and self-management skills).
- In orientation of nurse managers, address the shift from the nurse role at the bedside, and explain how to maintain the line of sight and create boundaries.

Clearly, socialization—the guided transition of a nurse manager into the new role—is a necessary, but not sufficient, component of building nurse manager engagement. Nurse manager sustainment must also be cultivated to prevent stagnation and to promote growth, skill attainment, accomplishment, and an ongoing sense of purpose. A number of approaches can promote engagement through sustainment:

- Create opportunities for ongoing contact with a mentor.
- Provide access to coaching and curriculum to address emotional mastery issues.
- Generate a continuing education plan that recognizes the developmental learning needs of long-time managers.
- Facilitate peer-mentor networks.
- Support self-renewal and activities to create balance and recharge the batteries of unit leaders (e.g., flex schedules, gym memberships, meal vouchers, opportunities to attend conferences and order room service).

TRANSFORMING CULTURES FOR ENGAGEMENT

Cultures of engagement can be designed and built through deliberate strategies. These strategies include transformation of cultural values and key relationships, graduate and continuing education, orientation/training and sustainment education of nurse managers, interviewing and personnel decisions, job descriptions and use of the recruitment system, and organizational self-study and development. The Nurse Manager Engagement Questionnaire (NMEQ) is a qualitative interview tool that health organizations can use to nurture both line of sight and mission alignment.

Cultivate a Learning Culture

- Assess different learning needs for initiation and sustainment of nurse managers.
- Provide a formal orientation process.

- Support a peer network through formal education and graduate degree work.
- Provide new nurse managers with a book of knowledge, including information about both the clinical and psychological aspects of the role.
- Provide ongoing clinical and emotional education.
- Encourage growth by introducing new experiences, risks, and challenges that carry managers beyond their comfort level.
- Provide easy access to on-site learning.
- Create partnerships with educational institutions to provide on-site degree programs.
- Offer tuition loans and reimbursement.
- Encourage and underwrite educational conference attendance.

Build a Culture of Regard

- Educate staff nurses about the multifaceted aspects of the nurse manager role.
- Increase accountability, decision-making authority, and empowerment of managers.
- Facilitate more nurse–physician contact and collegial relationships through joint participation in task forces and projects and via joint rounding.
- Legitimize the evidence base that nurse managers provide in decision making.
- Recognize nurse managers' contributions by offering work–life balance incentives for rejuvenation (e.g., encourage vacation time and offer vouchers for massages, take-out dinners, tickets to events, and reduced health club membership fees).
- Create cultural rituals of recognition and rejuvenation.

Craft a Culture of Meaning

- Design annual line of sight surveys that map how managers spend their time and that underline how nurse managers' work contributes to meeting the goals of patient care and supporting the organization's goals and values.
- Include discussion of questions from the NMEQ (e.g., managers' high point experiences, generative moments, and contributions) in all performance evaluation sessions.

- Remove obstacles that block nurse managers' line of sight to the results of patient care. Reconfigure their workload by adding additional personnel (e.g., a clinical instructor or business assistant).

Develop a Culture of Generativity

- Introduce the word generativity into the organization to create a shared language, which symbolizes a culture shift.
- Take the capacity for generativity into account in job descriptions, succession planning, talent management, and job interviews.
- Designate, recognize, and reward mentors as part of both the socialization and sustainment processes.
- Create cultural rituals (e.g., awards and recognition programs) to highlight storytelling about mentors and acts of generativity.
- Include mentorship and generative behavior as part of performance evaluation for every position.
- Create coaching/mentoring labs that include role-playing.
- "Manage by walking around" to increase availability.
- Remove organizational obstacles to the manager's access to senior leadership for coaching and consultation.

Establish a Culture of Excellence

- Cultivate organizational esteem through communication about accomplishments, grants, research, patient satisfaction scores, and success stories.
- Communicate with clarity about standards of excellence and benchmarks; celebrate their completion or achievement.

THE FUTURE OF ENGAGEMENT

The original Nurse Manager Engagement Project (NMEP), which was funded by the Robert Wood Johnson Foundation, addressed the urgent dilemma of nursing shortages by detailing the qualities and experiences of successful long-term nurse managers and their organizations. In this study, retention was used as a metric, rather than a model. The results yielded promising exemplary models of nurse manager engagement, along with a significant number of possible strategies for enhancing excellence and longevity.

In the years since the study was completed, these dimensions of engagement have resonated in many classrooms and conversations. The future of engagement—or so the smart kids tell us—is that engaged nurse managers will, in turn, contribute to retention and engagement of staff nurses. In the meantime, consider the marching orders from Cynthia J., a TCAB nurse manager from Indiana. She wrote:

> Middle managers need to understand the importance of their role as innovators in keeping a healthy work environment. Teamwork takes respect for self and others. Reinvest in ongoing educating and training of staff and self. Embrace risk taking and small tests of change that support safe, timely, efficient, effective, equitable, and patient-centered care. Find joy in small things. Know that passion, love, and compassion are very powerful in the way things get done in health care when it is directed to the bedside.

By playing it forward, managers like Cynthia will develop into the once and future leaders of their organizations.

References

Adams, J. (2005). *Boundary intelligence*. Hoboken, NJ: John Wiley and Sons.

Aiken, L. H., & Patrician, P. A. (2000). Measuring organizational traits of hospitals: The revised nursing work index. *Nursing Research, 49*, 46–153.

Bassi, L., & McMurrer, D. (2007). Maximizing your return on people. *Harvard Business Review*, 1–10.

Bennis, W. (1989). *Why leaders can't lead*. San Francisco: Jossey-Bass.

Bird, W. A. (2001). *A comparison of positive outcome expectancies*. Unpublished doctoral research paper, Biola University, La Mirada, CA.

Borchardt, C. (2005). Creating passion through a supportive practice environment. *Nurse Leader, 3*(5), 31–35.

Boswell, W., & Boudreau, J. (2004). How "line of sight" helps with "big picture": How do you view your firm? *Human Resource Management International Digest, 129*(3), 15–17.

Bradley, C., Marcia, L., & James, E. (1998, February). Generativity and stagnation: A five category model. *Journal of Personality, 66*(1), 39–64.

Bunsey, S., DeFazio, L. L. B., & Jones, S. (1991). Nurse managers: Role expectations and job satisfaction. *Applied Nursing Research, 4*, 7-1.

Burnard, P. (1992). Learning from experience: Nurse tutors' and student nurses' perceptions of experiential learning in nurse education: Some initial findings. *International Journal of Nursing Studies, 29*(2), 151–161.

Byrne, M. W., & Keefe, M. R. (2002). Building research competence in nursing through mentoring. *Journal of Nursing Scholarship, 34*(4).

Cooke, R., & Lafferty, J. (1989). *Organization culture inventory*. Plymouth, MI: Human Synthesis.

Cooke, R. A., & Rosseau, D. M. (1988). Behavioral norms and expectations: A quantitative approach to the assessment of organizational culture. *Group and Organization Studies, 13*(3), 245–248.

Cooperrider, D. (1990). *Appreciative management and leadership: The power of positive thought and action in organizations*. San Francisco: Jossey-Bass.

Cooperrider, D. (1995). *Introduction to appreciative inquiry: Organizational development* (5th ed.). New York: Prentice Hall.

De Burca, S. (2000). The learning healthcare organization. *International Journal for Quality in Healthcare, 12*(6), 457–458.

Edmondson, A. (1996). Learning from mistakes is easier said than done: Group and organizational influences on the detection and correction of human error. *Journal of Applied Behavioral Science, 32*(1), 5–28.

Erikson, E. H. (1950). *Childhood and society.* New York: Norton.

Firth, K. (2002). Leadership: Balancing the clinical and managerial roles. *Professional Nursing, 17*(8), 486–489.

Fletcher, C. (2001). Hospital RNs' job satisfactions and dissatisfactions. *Journal of Nursing Administration, 31*(6), 324–326.

Freud, A. (1937). *The ego and the mechanisms of defense.* London: Hogarth Press.

Galinsky, M., & Moskowitz, G. (2000). Perspective taking: Decreasing stereotype expression, stereotype accessibility and in-group favoritism. *Journal of Psychology and Personality, 74*(4), 70–74.

Gladwell, M. (2009). *Outliers: The story of success.* Boston: Little, Brown.

Goleman, D. (1995). *Emotional intelligence: Why it can matter more than IQ.* New York: Bantam Books.

Goleman, D. (1998a, November–December). What makes a leader? *Harvard Business Review,* 93–102.

Goleman, D. (1998b). *Working with emotional intelligence.* New York: Bantam Books.

Grandey, A. (2000). Emotional regulation in the workplace: A new way to conceptualize emotional labour. *Journal of Occupational Health Psychology, 5*(1), 95–110.

Gratton, L., & Ghoshol, S. (2005). Beyond best practices. *Sloan Management Review, 46,* 49–57.

Gubman, E. (2004). From engagement to passion for work: The search for the missing person. *Human Resource Planning, 27.*

Hartmann, E. (1991). *Boundaries in the mind: A new psychology of personality.* New York: Basic Books.

Heifetz, R., & Linksky, M. (2002). *Leadership on the line.* Cambridge, MA: Harvard Business School Press.

Husserl, E. (1999). *The essential Husserl,* ed. D. Weton. Bloomington: Indiana University Press.

Ickes, W. (1997). *Empathic accuracy.* New York: Guilford Press.

John, C. (2004). *Becoming a reflective practitioner.* Oxford, UK: Blackwell.

John, C., & Freshwater, D. (1986). *Transforming nursing through reflective practice.* Oxford, UK: Blackwell.

Kahn, W. (1990). Psychological conditions of personal engagement and disengagement at work. *Academy of Management Journal, 33*(4), 692–724.

Kanter, R. (1993). *Men and women of the corporation.* New York: Basic Books.

Kegan, R. (1983). *The evolving self.* Cambridge, MA: Harvard University Press.

Kegan, R. (2002). *How the way we talk can change the way we work: Seven languages for transformation.* New York: John Wiley and Sons.

Kerfoot, K. (1998). Management is taught, leadership is learned. *Plastic Surgical Nursing, 18*(2), 108–110.

King, T. (1999). Scanning and reflecting: Major components of nursing leadership. *Health Care for Women International, 20*(3), 315–323.

Kotre, J. (1984). *Outliving the self: Generativity and the interpretation of lives.* Baltimore: Johns Hopkins University Press.

Kouzes, J., & Posner, B. (2003). *The leadership challenge.* San Francisco: Jossey-Bass.

Kramer, M., & Schmalenberg, C. (1988). Magnet hospitals: Part I: Institutions of excellence. *Journal of Nursing Administration, 18*(1), 13–24.

Kramer, M., & Schmalenberg, C. (2003). Securing good nurse–physician relationships. *Nursing Management, 34*(7), 34–38.

Laschinger, H., & Purd, N. (2007). Antecedents and consequences of nurse managers' perceptions of organizational support. *Nursing Economics, 24*(1), 20–29.

Leigh-Edward, K., & Gylo-Hercelinsky, J. (2007). Burnout in the caring nurse: Resilient behaviors. *British Journal of Nursing, 16*(4), 240–242.

Leigh-Edward, K., & Warelow, P. (2005). Resilience: When coping is emotionally intelligent. *Journal of the American Psychiatric Nurses Association, 11*(2), 101–102.

Mackoff, B., & Wenet, G. (2004). *The inner work of leaders: Leadership as a habit of mind.* New York: Amacom.

Manion, J. (2005). Supporting nurse managers in creating a culture of retention. *Nurse Leader, 2,* 52–56.

McAdams, D. P., & de St. Aubin, E. (1992). A theory of generativity and its assessment through self-report, behavioral acts, and narrative themes in autobiography. *Journal of Personality and Social Psychology, 62,* 1003–1015.

McAdams, D. P., Hart, H., & Maruna, S. (1998). The anatomy of generativity. In D. P. McAdams & E. de St. Aubin (Eds.), *Generativity and adult development: How and why we care for the next generation.* Washington, DC: APA Press.

Mills, C. (2005). Developing the ability to lead. *Nursing Management, 12*(4), 20–23.

Musselwhite, W. C., & Ingram, R. P. (1995). *Change style indicator.* NC: Discovery Learning.

Olson, R. (Ed.). (2002). *The mentor connection in nursing.* New York: Springer.

Ormond, L. (1994). Developing emotional insulation. *International Journal of Group Psychotherapy, 44,* 5.

Parsons, M., & Stonestreet, J. (2003). Factors that contribute to nurse manager retention. *Nursing Economics, 21,* 120–126.

Parsons, M. L., & Cornett, P. A. (2006). Creating healthy workplaces: Laying the groundwork by listening to nurse managers. *Nurse Leader, 4*(3), 34–39.

Patrick, A., & Spence-Laschinger, H. (2006). The effect of structural empowerment and perceived organizational support on middle level nurse managers' role satisfaction. *Journal of Nursing Management, 14*(1), 13–16.

Piaget, J. (1983). *The moral judgment of the child.* Harmondsworth, UK: Penguin Books.

Rhoades, L., & Eisenberger, R. (2001). Affective commitment to the organization: The contribution of perceived organizational support. *Journal of Applied Psychology, 86,* 825–836.

Robinson, D., & Perryman, S. (2004). *The drivers of employee engagement.* UK: Institute for Employee Studies, IES Report 408, pp. 3–5.

Salovey, P., & Mayer, J. (1990). Emotional intelligence imagination. *Cognition and Personality, 9*(3), 185–211.

Salovey, P., & Mayer, J. (1997). *Emotional development and emotional intelligence: Educational implications.* New York: Basic Books.

Scheier, M., & Carver, C. (1992). The effects of optimism on psychological and physical well-being. *Cognitive Therapy and Research, 16,* 201–228.

Schon, D. A. (1987). *Educating the reflective practitioner.* San Francisco: Jossey-Bass.

Seligman, M. (1992). *Learned optimism.* New York: Pocket Books.

Selman, R. (1980). The emotionally intelligent workplace. In *The growth of interpersonal understanding: Developmental and clinical analyses.* New York: Academic Press.

Shanock, S., & Eisenberger, R. (2006). Relationships with subordinates' perceived supervisor support, perceived organizational support and performance. *Journal of Applied Psychology, 91,* 689–695.

Silverman, M. (2002). The will to succeed and the capacity to do so: The power of positive identifications. *Psychoanalytic Quarterly, 71,* 777–800.

Silvettin, C. (2000). Where will tomorrow's nurse managers come from? *Journal of Nursing Administration, 32,* 185–188.

Spence-Laschinger, H., & Finegan, J. (2005). Using empowerment to build trust and respect in the workplace. *Nursing Economics, 23,* 6–13.

Srsic-Stoehr, K., & Rogers, L. (2004). Success skills for the nurse manager: Cultural debut and sustainment. *Nurse Leader, 2*(6), 36–41.

Sternin, J. (2003). Practice positive deviance for extraordinary social and organizational change. In L. Carter, D. Ulrich, & M. Goldsmith (Eds.), *The change champion's field guide* (pp. 20–37). New York: Best Practice Publications.

Stewart-Amidei, C. (2003, April). A culture of excellence. *Journal of Neuroscience Nursing, 35*(2).

Sullivan, J., Bretschnieder, J., & McCausland, M. (2003). Designing a leadership development program for nurse managers' evidence driven approach. *Journal of Nursing Administration, 33*(1), 544–549.

Tart, C. (1975). *States of consciousness.* New York: Dutton.

Vaillant, G. (1993). *The wisdom of the ego.* Cambridge, MA: Harvard University Press.

Vitello-Cicciu, J. (2003). Innovative leadership through emotional intelligence. *Nursing Management, 34*(10), 28–32.

Wagner, R., & Harter, J. (2006). *12: The elements of great managing.* New York: Gallup Press.

Walker, R. (2006, July 30). The brand underground. *New York Times*, pp. 1–7.

Watkins, K. E., & Marsick, V. J. (1993). *Sculpting the learning organization.* San Francisco: Jossey-Bass.

West, W. (1994). Learning organizations: A critical review. In L. Martin (Ed.), *Proceedings of the Midwest Research-to-Practice Conference.* Madison: University of Wisconsin.

Whyte, D. (2001). *Crossing the unknown sea: Work as a pilgrimage of identity.* New York: Riverbooks.

Wilson, V. (2005). Mentorship: Developing and inspiring the next generation of leaders. *Nurse Leader, 3*(6), 44–66.

Zillmann, D. (1993). Mental control of angry aggression. In D. Wegner & J. Pennebaker (Eds.), *Handbook of mental control.* Upper Saddle River, NJ: Prentice Hall.

Glossary

Affirmative framework: A consistent way of thinking defined by the use of a positive explanatory style and the capacity to envision and anticipate positive outcomes.

Appreciative inquiry: A research and solution-based model, created by organizational psychologist David Cooperrider, that is grounded in the practice of asking unconditionally positive questions to imagine and build on the positive core of a person or an organization.

Ardor: A quality evidenced as a heightened emotional connection to work and a deep investment in patient care and commitment to the organization.

Attunement: A quality characterized by regard for the contribution of each person in the organization and setting aside assumptions to understand diverse perspectives.

Boundary clarity: The capacity to connect with others without losing a sense of self.

Bracketing: The phenomenologist and philosopher Edmond Husserl's term for setting aside assumptions to gain a broader perspective.

Change agility: An ability marked by comfort with change, capacity for innovation, and the desire for new learning challenges.

Culture of excellence: An organization that communicates high standards and expectation of excellence and cultivates brand pride in its accomplishments and reputation.

Culture of generativity: An organization that nurtures the next generation through visible and approachable role models and deliberate mentoring relationships.

Culture of meaning: An organization that is distinguished by clarity about its mission and values and the alignment of individual and organizational goals and priorities.

Culture of regard: An organization that conveys regard for nursing through responsiveness to viewpoints and decisions of nurses, collegial nurse–physician relationships, and facilitation of the attainment of nursing goals.

Emotional insulation: A term used by psychiatrist Louis Ormond to describe the creation of an internal boundary that allows experience in, but protects the self from being overwhelmed by negative emotions in self or others.

Emotional mastery: A set of emotional tools for managing the unique challenges of the nurse manager role, including reflection, boundary clarity, self-regulation, attunement, change agility, and an affirmative framework.

Engagement: A model for the heightened emotional connection that an employee feels for the organization—one that influences the employee to work with superior productivity, job performance, and longevity.

Ethos: The characteristic spirit and sentiments of a people or community.

Explanatory style: Psychologist Martin Seligman's term for what you say to yourself about how you explain challenging events.

Generativity: Psychologist Erik Erickson's term for the ability to find gratification in the development of others, creating a legacy in one's image, linking generations, and offering autonomy and power to the next generation.

Identification: A manager's capacity to see his or her own achievement in the success of the manager's staff and in creating an atmosphere for superb care.

Learning culture: An organization identified by abundant opportunities for continuing education, learning through risk taking, and transparency of information and resources.

Line of sight: Described by researchers Wendy Boswell and John Boudreau, the way an individual understands how his or her day-to-day work contributes to the larger vision, values, and objectives of the organization.

Mission driven: Characterized by orientation to purpose, big-picture thinking, and a focus on end results, while still addressing day-to-day concerns.

Nurse Manager Engagement Questionnaire (NMEQ): A self-report survey instrument that can be used to elicit data about individual and organizational behaviors linked to nurse manager engagement.

Positive deviance: An applied research approach, developed by organizational innovator Jerry Sternin, that emphasizes studying and adopting the "uncommon" strategies of people in the community who have solved a common problem.

Reflection: The capacity to leverage lessons from experience, and to observe the effects of one's own behavior on others.

Retention: A metric for commitment to one's job, measured by amount of time on the job or employed by the organization.

Scanning: A term used by nurse educator Ti King to describe the practice of searching for cues about self and others and reflecting on these cues to enhance communication.

Self-regulation: The capacity to manage and regulate internal states, thoughts, speech, and actions to achieve organizational and individual goals.

Signature behaviors: The factors that embody positive values, characteristics, aspirations, and interests of individuals and their organizations.

Socialization of nurse managers: The education and support required to successfully guide the transition of a staff nurse into a nurse manager role.

Sustainment: The training and support required to foster replenishment and commitment in long-term staff and managers.

Transcript of Full Interview

All identifiers have been removed to protect confidentiality. Consider the perspectives of a nurse manager of 5 ½ years who backed into the job when two units were combined. She demonstrates her agility with change—she's a unit fixer. Pay close attention to how she reframed what it means to care for patients as a manager and how she maintained strong boundaries with patients, families, and staff. She is keyed to listen and identify the deeper process and meaning in a patient or staffer's words. Note her unique way of side stepping negativity, transforming reactive people and situations into to responsive ones.

Use this interview transcript for your own research as a case study or as a discussion focus in class. As you read, try to identify the signature strengths of the individual nurse manager being interviewed as well as the strengths of her organization.

B = Interviewer

P = Participant

B: I want to start with the beginnings of your nurse manager role, which was 5½ years ago. Tell me about the first few weeks and months—any positive impressions or promising things that happened during that time.

P: I think initially I felt very welcomed into the role. I was actually approached for the role. It's not something I actively looked for; it was not an opportunity that arose when our current unit director, who I had worked with for about four or five months, decided to step down. It was a newer unit in the sense that it was moved from [name omitted] Hospital across from the stem cell transplant unit—so it was a newer unit that was a combined staff from [name omitted].

It was at a time when a group of people came together who didn't know each other, and a unit that was significantly short staffed. I looked at it as an opportunity to advance my career. Initially [I] was approached [as if the new position were] more like a permanent charge nurse role, where I would be there Monday through Friday. My idea of the job was being a permanent charge nurse, rallying with the doctors, and looking at staffing day-to-day—not realizing it's going into the whole other HR piece of it, the whole gimmick. I think what made it positive in the beginning was the help other people provided. I didn't feel isolated. It was not my clinical director at the time, [but rather] more the peer group of unit directors that was most helpful.

B: So a peer group of directors of other units. Tell me a little bit about what you remember about them: Was it any particular person? What are some sort of scenarios from that?

P: Anytime I had a question, I could pick up the phone. There were certain unit directors who were good at certain things. If I didn't know how to do something with the scheduling system that we had, there was a certain individual I could call for that; if it was a payroll question, it was a different person. We just focused on who had the strength in what areas. One person wasn't your contact.

B: Who was your "go to" person? How did you know the "go to" people?

P: From the unit director who was on the sister oncology unit. She knew who to call; if she did not know the answer, she would refer me to that person. I was given a list of "who does this well." [The director would say,] "I don't know how to help with that. Why don't you call this person?" When you realize which unit directors had the strengths in which areas, it seemed to help.

B: So, early on you discovered that there was one person who really knew who to go to. And when you did go to those people, they were really helpful and had what you were looking for.

P: Right. They were helpful.

B: The way that you describe it, you took on a leadership role and [you thought] you knew [what] it was, but what it actually turned out to be was a much bigger role than you thought. Tell me a little bit about that and what you thought when you realized, "This is a big job."

P: What I wanted to do with the role, I wanted to continuously round. Initially I started rounding with the doctors every day, but as the role developed for me, I realized that was not feasible. The thing that would be a downside for me is I felt that I lost a lot of patient contact. We do daily rounds now, which kind of facilitates that.

B: How is the job different from what you thought it would be? You thought it would be at least at the core of rounding with physicians.

P: I think the HR piece—looking at a unit that was significantly understaffed and knowing that my biggest challenge was getting a unit staffed [for] a higher-acuity unit; looking at taking in graduate nurses and how that affected [the staffing]. In my stem cell transplant background, we never hired graduate nurses into [the unit]. This is where we started doing it—[it was a first] for me in my career. That is when I realized that what I thought the job was and what the job actually was, were two different things.

B: So it was that hiring aspect, and particularly hiring from a pool that you hadn't used previously in this field. What did you think about that?

P: I was willing to take it on because at the time if I didn't, I never would have hired enough people to get the unit up and running. The next year I hired 21 nurses in one year, the majority of whom were graduate nurses. I think there were a handful of experienced nurses, and their oncology experience was minimal in comparison to what I was used to.

B: During that early time, what seemed like a sign or a positive anticipation of the role? One of the things you pointed to earlier is that you thought there would be more patient contact directly and through rounds, and then it turned out to be not so much. How did you come to peace with that?

P: I think it was a sense of accomplishment that I took a unit that was completely short staffed and made it so it worked. We were no longer considered the shortest-staffed unit in the hospital. We were getting a group of very seasoned senior nurses mixed with a very inexperienced group of nurses.

B: I am very intrigued with this whole idea of you coming into the field and even into the position with the idea that it is about patient contact and imagining yourself rounding with physicians, and then finding out it's a whole lot of other stuff. [Do you find your responsibilities gratifying enough to be a substitute for patient contact?] How does that work for you?

P: I don't think it substituted. I think that when I realized that the patients need the staff, I was still playing a key role in taking care of these patients. . . . [In] my beginning days, [I] didn't know the patient satisfaction scores . . . , but my understanding was that the unit had a low patient satisfaction [and we have reached] the point now that we have the highest patient satisfaction. [I feel good] knowing that along the way, my role—although I don't want to say it is minor because I think it is major—[helped] get these nurses from where we were low to where we are high now.

B: So in a way it's like a reframe: "I am doing patient care."

P: Right. Not actually physically taking care of [patients] but providing the staff to take care of them.

B: If you couldn't have made that switch, it would have been difficult because of what you came in with—you wanted to take care of patients and you wanted to do rounds. How do you think it made that shift, because it really fascinates me that you could do that?

P: I don't know, because I still . . . miss taking care of patients [on a day-to-day basis.] From a clinical standpoint, I love to take care of patients, but I still find the position gratifying because I'm still in the role.

B: What do you say to the part of you that wants to take care of the patients?

P: I do from time to time. Usually it's when I take care of patients it's usually we know how to call off, I do it enough that it maintains that piece of it.

B: So you find a way to do that. State some ways that you found to stay in touch with the clinical aspect of caring for patients.

P: With any new things that come on board, I make sure that I try to attend the in-services as much as possible. I am in pretty much constant contact with my advanced practice nurse. She and I actually do all of the nursing orientation for our nurses. She is the primary contact for them, but I do meet with them. We meet with them on a weekly basis, 40 hours of shift work, so I stay kind of close that way. New chemotherapy regimens that we are doing—they are not new regimens, they are just new to our units. [I make] sure that I know what to expect with those regimens for the nursing staff. I still participate in our "train-the-trainer" [sessions] for chemotherapy administration. We have certain nurses who are responsible for training the nursing staff on the unit, so I am still familiar from that standpoint. And then I just take care of patients when the need arises. I don't preschedule it; I do it enough when we are short staffed on the unit.

B: You would step in so you still have your hand in on patient care. When you think back to your early time as a nurse manager, can you think of anything that you have learned that has helped you succeed in the years that followed?

P: I thought about that one a lot. [The first thing is that I don't take] things personally when people are upset. I think that was one of the hardest things for me in the beginning. If I could not get over that, I would have never stayed in the role. [If I had taken] every negative thing people have to say about the unit or what's going on . . . as a personal attack, I would have never survived. I have come a long way from that aspect. The second piece is listening to the staff. I listen to what they think would make something better. In the beginning, I was doing it all, like "We are going to do it this way." But I realized that did not build [my staff] as a team; it kind of made them fight against me. If I listened to them and adapted something that they wanted to do but still was in accordance with the hospital [policy], then it worked better.

B: You learned to be more of a collaborator with the staff, but also there's a key aspect that deals with valuing their information or their points of view. And the first part about not taking it personally—many people would like to know how you did that. You do hear that refrain in nursing because you deal with so many different people who can get angry or upset with something about policy, process, or what is going on for them or the family. Can you reconstruct in any way how you learned how to do that?

P: I think it just came through experience from a patient perspective. Usually it was not patients; it was more the family. If I had a family who was very dissatisfied with some aspect of the hospitalization, it was not always related to the nursing care, [although] at times it was. As time goes by, it seems like they are very happy with the nursing care. But there's other aspects of the admission. . . . [W]hen you're looking at this patient and family, is it actually the scenario that's going on with that patient? Is it an end-of-life issue or is the patient going downhill slowly over a period of time, and how much is that impacting what they are dissatisfied with? This is [the family's] way to forget about that: "I am going to complain because this is going to make me feel better."

With staff, a lot of times I found out at the end when I did take it personally they really weren't mad; it was not a personal attack. It was just "I'm angry about this scenario." There were times that the decisions I made did affect them. I can think of a very clear example—when I wanted to do scheduling the way I did it when I was a staff nurse where I worked. I was part of the scheduling committee, but I didn't make the decisions, and I thought as a staff nurse I was very satisfied with [the system]. I was a lower person on the seniority pole; I wasn't a high-seniority person. . . . I felt that the holiday schedule worked very well where you just rotated Christmas and New Year's every year: If you work Christmas Eve and Christmas Day, you were off New Year's Eve and New Year's Day, and you just rotated each year. One year I made the decision: "This is how we are going to do it." I made a lot of people angry, especially the senior staff. The less senior staff were very happy. My mix was mostly less seasoned staff and more inexperienced staff, so they were very happy with [the scheduling,] but my very senior staff were very angry about it. I learned through that. Personally, I don't think they were attacking me; it was the idea that they had to work Christmas.

There was never a manager who told them they had to do that before. So I did adapt. I adapted it so that they could choose the holiday, and we moved people based on seniority but would not move the same people every year.

B: The way you're able to not take it personally with the patients and their families is to always be aware of what their actual situation is—that they might be taking those feelings and projecting them onto you. You just keep in mind as you are responding that it's not about you, it's how they feel about everything else and what they are thinking about everything else. And then with staff, [the bad feelings are] often directed toward a decision you made—which isn't the same as you.

P: Yes. With staff, it's very hard, because sometimes I think that their personal life relates. I think your personal life and your work life affect each other. If things aren't going well in your personal life, your way to deal with that sometimes is being angry with everything at work, or being an excellent clinical provider at this point. I think it depends on the individuals being able to figure out the real thing that they are angry about.

B: Right. That's not dissimilar to what you describe with patients and their families. So those are largely learnings over those years. How would explain the positive factors that have influenced your decision to stay at your job for 5½ years?

P: Scheduling is one. I think that I do have flexibility with my own personal scheduling. It works very well. My husband also works in health care. The way we take care of our children is that I come in early, and we're usually here around 6:00 in the morning. I'm a morning person so that's no problem for me. [It] used to be I always left by 3:30. I don't leave now until 4:35. My days are starting to get longer and longer, which has been somewhat of a [source of dissatisfaction] over the past 6 to 7 months, but I'm trying to manage my time a little bit differently. I'm looking at the best way to manage time. There is flexibility, and if I do need to leave before 3:30 or 4:30, I can. I am able to do that as long as I have the appropriate coverage for me. It works out well. My husband and I both are home late in the evening together. So scheduling is one aspect.

It's also important for me that I take—and I never used to be a vacation person—but I would make sure to take at least three whole-week vacations every year, whether that is leaving the city or just having time off away from work. What I'm realizing now is that it might be important to have a few more days off in between [those vacation weeks.] I tend not to take days off; I usually just work until I take a week off and then that's it. I'm trying to figure out how to balance that so it is flexible from that standpoint.

B: What are other positive things that have helped you and influenced you to stay in the role as nurse manager here?

P: It's been something that has been challenging. There is always something new that I have learned. I don't think it really matters how many years I have been here, there is always some HR [issue] that I didn't know existed. Being in [this position] for five years, I have realized that staffing is an up-and-down roller coaster. When I first started, I thought I would never get out of the hole of being short staffed. Once you do get out of the hole, you realize that people do come and they do go, no matter how hard you try to retain them. You know you are going to get it fixed again. . . . My clinical director was a newer clinical director for me. I mean she wasn't the first to put me in this role; it was a different clinical director at the time. But I remember that there was a peer unit director who had a really short-staffed unit, and she was going on and on about how horrible it was. I just looked at her and I said, "You know, I was at that point two years ago and there is a light at the end of the tunnel. You just have to keep hiring; they will be there." I remember my clinical director saying, "That was the best thing that you could have said to her"—instead of what a lot of directors do, they tend to just go on about how negative it is. When you do that, it doesn't help.

There is a group here that gets together on a regular basis. I have gone there a few times, but all they do is complain and that brings me down. That is one thing that keeps me in the role—I try to stay away from the negativity piece of it. If I listen to everybody else complain, I will start to become negative, so if I stay away from it, I do best.

B: So it's a conscious choice to think resiliently and to not spend a lot of time in the company with people who do not.

P: Right.

B: That's a positive about you, that you have made this decision. Is there anything else about this place or the role that has allowed you to stay?

P: I don't know the answer to that. It's curious because I was thinking when they asked me to do this [interview], it kind of shocked me. I have been here for five years, and I didn't realize that! I honestly didn't; I don't count off the years. But then I looked at the other questions they were asking, and I got to thinking, "I am one of the top as far as years of service in the unit director group when you start looking at who is in that role." Then I started wondering, "Why is everybody leaving?" I honestly don't know the answer to that question, because I don't participate in that negativity.

B: That's what the question is—why do you stay? You said it's challenging and you personally avoid the negativity. What else keeps you here?

P: I like the idea of being the unit director from a professional standpoint. I love being a nurse; foremost, I love being a nurse. It was the best career for me. But I still feel being a unit director, I am able to see that in my staff.

B: How would you put it? What do you see in your staff?

P: The staff that I have is a group that delivers care compassionately. They have demonstrated that through the high patient satisfaction scores that we have. We do see a group of patients over and over again. One of the things that is depressing is taking care of a lot of leukemia patients who don't make it, and we see the bulk of that. We don't see all the ones who are doing very well. I have worked with this staff to develop programs on how to deal with that aspect of [the nursing job]—you know, "This is what you can do." Everybody has an individual way of dealing with it. I run a few programs here and there that try to focus on what might help this group, but there is another group and there are some other programs that we try to run to help [nurses] as a retention aspect. I think just the idea that patients want to come, they want to be here—even though they don't want to be here, if they had to pick, this is where they want to be.

B: That is a real positive—to have created a place where people are seeking care. When you say you love nursing and it was the best career choice you could have made, and you see that in your nurses, what does that mean?

P: When I was a brand-new nurse, I started with ten other people around the same time. I was "the new nurse" for eight years, so I never saw anybody become a new nurse; I didn't see the progression.

B: You were the new kid on the block.

P: I was for eight years, yes. One of the things that my clinical director talked to me about, she said, "What are you doing for retention?" I said to her, I worked on a unit where the retention had to have been high; I worked there for eight years. Granted, it was during the time they were laying off nurses, too—there was an aspect of that. If you can believe, that was back in 1993 or 1994. We lost about three or four nurses off our unit because of [layoffs]. I tried to figure out what made that unit stay together and I don't know. I've tried and I don't know if it was because I was there for eight years and I just kind of got used to it.

B: It's hard. Could you point to any factors that kept it together?

P: I think we worked well as a team; that is one aspect. Whenever there was a nurse who was drowning in her day, someone was always there to help her out.

B: Drowning in her day?

P: Drowning in her day, like too many things to do that she couldn't keep on top of it.

B: Oh, yes, that's an amazing expression—but yes, that's really what it's like.

P: That's what I call it. I always say, "Let them drown a little bit." You know, with new nurses, I want to see if they are going to make it off of orientation. As a preceptor, [you need] to step back and let somebody try to fix [a problem] themselves before you jump in and save them. Then you know if they are able to get out of [the situation]. But that is very, very hard for any preceptor to do. [I enjoy] just watching [new nurses] go from "I know nothing as a nurse" to where they are in two years; I see big changes in 6 months, 1 year, 1½ to 2 years. One to two years is kind of where you decide whether this person is truly an oncology nurse.

B: The question I asked you was to follow up on the idea of "I love nursing"; I see that, and all of this is about the answer to the question of which positive factors have kept you here. Some of those positive factors are about you—so this is the next question, and it's a hard one. Which gifts and values and attributes and capabilities do you bring to this role that have helped you be successful? We were just talking about the fact that you are a deliberate, resilient thinker; [you also] avoid people who are not thinking that way and you try to refrain [from negative thinking]. You have that positive framework. Your colleague who was just here [in an earlier interview] said that it is so hard for nurses to talk about themselves. Given that, what would you say are your skills and capabilities and values that have allowed you to be successful?

P: I try to be a manager who works with the staff. Scheduling would be an example. I try to be very flexible with the scheduling; I know [nurses] have multiple reasons why they can't work certain days and certain schedules. I think being able to be flexible with them [is key]. If you don't, they are going to leave. If you can't balance their home life and their work life, one of them has to give, and 90% of the time (in my opinion) they are going to choose their family over their job. I feel that I am very flexible with scheduling. I am a very tough critic with time and attendance. [My nurses] all know that. I got feedback one time that they were fearful to call because it is an expectation that I get paged if they call in, so they have to call me.

They have been very good to me. After 10:00 P.M. and before 5:00 A.M., they don't call me. I got feedback from my clinical directors a couple of years ago about how I was not nice when [nurses] called off. [The director] said, "That's not a problem," but then I felt kind of bad. I don't want [nurses] *not* to call if they truly need to call. I am the one that they know will be there. In order for me to call off, there has to be something major going on, so I feel I am dependable from that standpoint. I think I'm flexible—again, maybe not with everything, but with scheduling and allowing [nurses] to work different kinds of shifts. It's not your traditional shifts; some of them work 16-hour shifts. I have nurses who live an hour away, so they work two [12-hour shifts] and a [16-hour shift.] I am able to give them the flexibility to do that.

Let's see, what else? This is hard. I think that I'm understanding of [nurses'] issues. I can't think that I resolve all of their issues, but I try to get those resolved for them.

B: Do you mean you can place yourself in their positions so you understand the situation and then comes the next part—which is what? Helping them strategize, figure out what to do?

P: I think one of the things about me is that I'm not a good problem solver, but I listen to what they think will solve it and then move from there and try to elaborate on that. I really can't offer anything else.

B: So it's more like for you, being understanding is providing companionship while somebody figures the problem out. They can talk out loud with you.

P: If they come up with the idea, I can show them how to get it moving.

B: So it's a collaborative process to do that. What else about you?

P: I think I have taken a team that was very highly reactive and turned them into being responsive.

B: Those are two interesting words, and I want to see how you define them. A team that was reactive is doing what?

P: They were very negative, they complained all the time, and they never looked happy when they came to work. Two years ago, I had patients complaining. The patients didn't like their nurses, and they didn't like the way they delivered their care. When I talk to patients now, they say, "I don't know if this is anything major to you; I think they are very good clinically, but what makes a difference is they come in with a smile." The nurses are cheerful and they want to meet the patients' needs. We all have bad days, but the majority of the nurses are smiling. They have moved away from the negativity and that took some terminations along the way. Some people left through a corrective action process, as part of following up on those issues that made them nurses you would not want on the unit.

B: You were able to shape an environment from its emotional climate. Those are some of the things you did strategically there. Do you think you are the type of person who can create a positive atmosphere?

P: Yes, over time. I don't think it is something that happens quickly. It took me two years to get there.

B: Yes, but to change the whole emotional climate is a big job. In some ways, it's a climate that is similar to your own [personality] in terms of approaching things in a more resilient way. Anything else you want to add?

P: I can't think of anything.

B: Let's turn this interview toward the cast of characters. There are so many people [in the hospital mix]—patients, physicians, families, staff, other colleagues, et cetera. What do you bring to the middle manager role that allows you to connect with so many different people?

P: I think it might be being able to balance all of them. I don't know if this is the right question for this answer. The one thing I always question is, "How do you balance your upper administration with your direct reports?" That is truly middle management. My father has always been in middle management. He has been in upper middle management for the most part. That is the question I asked him: "How do you balance the two?" If you make the upper-management people happy, sometimes it doesn't make your lower-level people happy, and vice versa. Being able to communicate and balance between the two is something I don't know how to do. I have tried, and I don't know if I am doing a good job of that. I find that the most difficult thing to do.

B: You have a desire of wanting to do that right but not always sure that you are doing it the right way?

P: Sometimes I agree with both sides. I can see both sides of it.

B: When you think of things that you do wisely or well in terms of communicating with different people, what do you think you do well?

P: I am a good listener. Over time, I have learned to ask the right question, to try to get to what they are really trying to tell me. [Here's an example:] If a patient says something such as, "I hear you are short staffed," I want to know exactly what they are getting at. Are they just hearing that, or do they truly feel that because there is an aspect of their care that they are not getting? Learning how to ask this [is important,] because before I would just respond by saying, "Oh no, we're not short staffed." Now I realize that there is some point beyond that and they are not saying it to me. I try to pull that information from them.

I have done that with staff, also. It was actually with a physician, but it included a staff member who was one of our fellows. They were complaining about our attending physicians not calling in the admissions, and I couldn't get out of [the physician] who and why. Finally, for some reason, I said to him, "Well, who is doing it?" He answered that question. So then I knew who was doing it and who was not doing it just by asking the question in a positive way. I have used that tool and I have gotten much better responses by using that aspect of it. I try to find the positive answer versus the negative answer depending on the scenario.

B: Can you think of anything else? It is interesting the way you describe your listening. Someone once said there is process listening and there is content listening. You listen for process. The question could be, "Are you are understaffed?" But you are looking for the process, such as "this person is afraid they are being ignored or if there is a crisis there will be no one to take care of them." When you listen in that kind of depth, it really gets you to what someone is really talking about and what their intentions are. That has proved to be a real communication key.

P: It's not something I knew five years ago; it is something I learned along the way—trying to figure out the root of what they are really talking about.

B: When you say, "This is something I learned along the way," do you feel there have been situations that have taught you that?

P: The one scenario was dealing with that physician and trying to figure out who was not doing something. It was just by chance that I found out. I told my clinical director about it and she said that was fantastic. I said it wasn't something I actively thought about; it just came out of my mouth. When I realized what results it got, I decided I was going to use it again. It hasn't worked in every scenario, but it has worked in multiple ones. That's just learning through the experience of doing things wrong. I have done many things wrong, and I have learned from doing things wrong.

For example, one of the first nurses I ever hired was a graduate nurse. She and I had a rocky road. She was one of your nurses who was highly emotional and took everything personally. In fact, this was similar to how I was when I was a new nurse. I could relate to her. When I look at her as a nurse now, she no longer works for me but is working in the outpatient department, and is currently moving with her family down south, but she came by to see patients the other day. I have known her for about five years.

I never would have thought that she would have turned out to be the type of nurse she is now, based on her first year. She told me a couple of years ago that she was always intimidated by me. I asked her if she was intimidated by the way I treated her or by the person I was. She said she didn't know. It made me think about how I could make new hires feel comfortable in coming to me. She said she never felt comfortable in coming to me when she was newly hired. She said, "You were my boss and I didn't want you to judge me." No matter how many times I told her that I was not judging her and I wanted her to come to me if she needed help, [she felt that way]. I have yet to figure out how to do that. I have had multiple people over the years. I think it is personal issues with individual people.

B: When you say you have had a number of people over the years, what do you mean? That they would come to you?

P: How to take a new employee, when you are the boss, how to eliminate the fact that they see you as a boss but not a peer. They still have to see you as boss.

B: You have a really good way of reflecting on your own behavior. There are boundary issues—for example, between upper management and staff—and you ask yourself how you would manage those issues. You do evaluate the staff, but you don't want them to feel judged. You want them to feel unconditional regard for you so that they can come to you when they have problems. I think we have to add to your strength column that you have a very keen, sort of third eye, about yourself. You don't despair about it. You really take these situations and learn from them. You have touched on this a little, but I want you to really direct some thought to this. What do you see as satisfying and gratifying about your experience as middle management in this setting and what do you contribute that gives you a feeling of pride?

P: One of the things that is my biggest accomplishment is the high patient satisfaction. That means a lot to me. I love my patients. Overall, that has been my biggest accomplishment and it is something that has been maintained.

Another one is that I took a unit that originally was opened for only 16 beds. Within the first month of me taking on the unit, it was opened up to 20 beds. I was not staffed for 16 patients, let alone staffed for 20 patients. In the first month there was a lot of negativity on the unit, but [I was] able to take a significantly short-staffed unit to a fully functional unit and feel good about the schedule I put out. I do know that it waxes and wanes, but [I like] just knowing there is a way that you can hire enough people, get them through orientation, and retain enough of them. I still had some people leave throughout those times, but [I was] able to get out of it. That was something I accomplished in the last five years, and it took me two years to do that. When I finally hired those 21 nurses, I asked myself how I would get them to work together as a team.

B: Do you hear a theme here about transforming negativity and taking charge of it?

P: I will get it. When they start talking negatively, or when you are in a meeting and all they are doing is being negative. They keep talking about what is wrong, but no one is asking, "What are we going to do about it?" Now, my staff does not react as negatively to most scenarios. They have some times when they are very negative. I feel we move them; they don't stay negative very long. They stay negative for 24 to 48 hours or a few days, and then we move them to the most positive side of it.

[One key issue is] balancing staffing for the unit. One of the things when I started out, our sister unit was always sending me staff because I could not staff the unit without them. Then it reversed, and now we are staffing their unit. As a manager, you know that you need to get them help, but you also understand that you are not shorting them—but you are because you are not doing your ideal staffing. How do you get them to realize that you both need to balance this and getting them to do that? They still complain about that.

B: The question is not, "What is wrong?" but "What do you want more of?" It's not so much about how to fix it, it is more, "What do you want?" Can you describe a high-point experience in this setting when you felt really engaged and alive?

P: As a manager?

B: Yes, in this role.

P: I would have to say the idea that I finally—I mean it's a little thing—I put out a schedule that was fully staffed and had no holes. It took a long time to get to that point. But feeling good knowing that if you had a call-off, you had people who would come in and work extra. I have about eight or nine of my staff who would come in and work extra shifts and come in when you have the greatest need. I can't think of any more of my accomplishments.

B: It's not really so much an accomplishment as it is a feeling. For you, one thing that comes to mind is the schedule. Because you came in with a certain idea, and over time it evolved. When you finally came up with a schedule that people were really happy with, that was a big deal to you because it required a lot of your time and effort.

P: Just knowing that you have the confidence level that you have a good schedule put out there. There weren't any holes in the schedule.

B: Any other specific experience that stands out when you were really engaged?

P: I think the one thing I did is [to bring] in a bereavement-type support group. I brought them in on two occasions to talk to the staff. We were having a lot of young patients pass away. I had newer staff who were not able to handle it. They came to me asking what they could do about it. I got the name of this organization, got approval, and brought them in. The staff still talks about it, even though it was about two years ago. We brought this group in and I let the entire staff that was there, plus people who came in extra, meet in my conference room. I took all of their phones; no one could get a call. I had a group of nursing students on the floor with me that day. I ran the whole floor without them. I let them just be in there with the bereavement group and talk about their feelings without me being present. I don't think they would have opened up as much. Don't get me wrong, I had people in there who gave me feedback. I gave them the opportunity to do that without me, but I also took them away from patient care for an hour. This was difficult from my standpoint. For me, that was difficult to do because I didn't want to be that person who did not know what was going on in there. But at the same time, the staff really appreciated it. They made those comments to the organization about me being supportive of this. They said I had given up the time for them to talk about this without being interrupted. It's something little.

B: No, I think it was huge because the message behind it was that you recognized they had strong feelings and you were responsive to their needs, even if it meant you ran the floor with student nurses. It also showed that you respected their privacy because you were not present.

P: I still had feedback from the people who were running it but not breaching the confidentiality, just an overview of what their issues were.

B: Also, it is satisfying because you went over your comfort zone of not knowing what was going on. The need was so strong for them.

P: I don't think they would have opened up, because I did that with other scenarios that were similar—not bringing in an organization [from outside,] but bringing people who worked here. That group was an outside group. I think that made a difference because [the participants] did open up more. All the other sessions I had done, I was usually present. My upper administrative leader always told me that I needed to be present. I said I didn't think they would open up as much if I were present. It made a difference. I kind of went against what I was told to do, but I decided I would try it anyhow.

B: Have you had an opportunity to collaborate with a staff nurse in a partnership where it made a difference in someone's care?

P: I think when you look at difficult patient scenarios or difficult family scenarios, an area probably three years ago—it was a weaker area of mine, but stepping up—the nurses want to do patient care conferences. The nurses are very good at coming up with their own solutions. Everybody needs to hear the same message. Working with them on those aspects, I think I could do a better job at that. I think it's something I need to do instead of having the nurse come in and say, "I think we need to do a patient care conference on this scenario." It should be me prompting that. I let them drive that, depending on how significant the scenario is. It's probably something I need to work on.

B: A form of collaborating is either to convene or to be present at the patient conference?

P: I don't want to be the one saying, "This is what you should do." I want them to come up with those solutions. Deep down, I know what they need to do, but a lot of times if I give them the direction to do that, then it is always me telling them what to do. I think they have those solutions in them; they just haven't vocalized them yet.

B: It's really almost emboldening them to try it out. There's that sort of thing about someone drowning in their day and letting them find out they can actually swim to less choppy waters. It's a metaphor.

P: Well, you look at that metaphor, and you look at your new nurse and your seasoned nurse being paired together, the preceptor/orientee relationship. If you don't do that, the first day out of orientation, they will do that. That day is the worst day for them. You need to give them a day when they are fresh out of orientation that they have their best day. If they don't, they are going to keep looking at it negatively. . . . That gives me an idea of whether they are really ready to come off of orientation. Can they bring themselves back out from that? You want to save them, you have to save them.

B: Can you tell me about a time when someone in senior management helped you succeed?

P: I think when I look at the clinical director who is my direct supervisor—this is the one who did not hire me, who initially met with me. She didn't know me very well, she knew who I was, she knew what unit I was on, but I don't think she knew me personally. She asked me what my orientation was like. She took the time to ask me about my orientation, what I learned and what didn't work. Initially, my clinical director, the one who hired me, really did not guide me that much. When I compared [her behavior] to how this one guided me, I didn't know the difference at the time [but] I felt very supported by her. She looked at me as a director instead of someone who had been in the role for a year and a half, and gave me the guidance over the three years that I have been with her. She has always been there by my side, but she knows what my strengths are. She will say to me, "I know that you know how to do this." She lets me go do it, and then I will follow back up with her. When there is something [where] I truly don't know what to do, she will step in and help me. I don't know how to describe that. It is kind of like your mother–daughter relationship. She lets me fly and then brings me back in when she needs to.

B: It sounds like the right balance for you.

P: For a while there, I felt she wasn't supporting me because she was focusing on the other unit directors. There were two new unit directors and I felt unsupported at one point. I said to her, "I feel like you are never up here; you are always over there." She said, "It's because I know you are doing a good job. I know that you know what you are doing." I think in the end I was questioning my ability and my confidence level. She had high confidence in me.

B: It's a vote of confidence, actually not being around. The next question is, do you have a mentor in this setting? Do you consider her a mentor?

P: Yes, in comparison to anybody else, yes.

B: For you, for someone to be your mentor, what is required for that?

P: Somebody whom I can trust. Someone whom I can go to anytime. Last week, we had multiple things going on. A couple of the patients we have on the unit right now are very stressful [cases]. I'll use that word because I can't really go into detail; it's a very stressful situation for me. On top of that, we had the computer system go down at the end of the week. A computer system that we have been using for six weeks went down.

I can go to [the clinical director] and vent for five minutes and get those frustrations out because if I don't, I'm going to blow up on the unit. I know I can call her and vent and in five minutes, I'll feel much better. I can then be a better manager. Just having someone that you can do that with [is important]. I don't feel I can do that within my peer group. I had one individual I thought I could do that with at one point, but she is no longer in that role. I can do that with my clinical director. I don't think she looks at it as not being a good manager but as having reached a [certain] point, and she knows when I have reached my point. I feel supported in that way because I think we all need that person whom we can go to, when you get to that point, just needing five minutes to vent. Then you can relook at the situation. She will reel me back in. She says, "Why don't you go do this now?" This is supportive in my mind.

B: Ultimately because you're a person who likes to figure out what to do, not just what is wrong. Would you call her and say you need to vent or do you just call her venting?

P: I would call her up and start reviewing the situation and say that I am kind of angry about it. I don't use the word "venting," but at the end of the conversation

I will say to her, "Thank you for listening. I needed to get this off my chest." I do it without using inappropriate comments.

B: Well you get to vent and then she helps you look at how to get back on track. That is a real hallmark of a mentor.

P: It helps. I think we all need to have that person whom we can go to, whom we trust enough to say, "I'm having a bad day." Believe me, she puts me in line or she will tell me when I'm not doing something right. She'll tell me when I'm wrong and will lead me. I think that's important, because as a manager you have to be able to support your staff but also tell them when they are not doing something right. She does that.

B: You can count on her for honesty. How has this particular organization been a good fit for you in terms of staying?

P: Initially when I came here, I didn't come here because of [name of hospital]; I came here because the doctors whom I worked for at another institution came here. I followed them. Mainly because the job I was working before, the doctors left with the whole oncology group and I felt that the unit where I worked was going to general medical/surgical and I wanted my leukemia patients. I love taking care of leukemia patients. That is the main reason I came here. There was no other reason for me leaving the other institution.

In the years that I have been here, I have always felt supported by upper management. I feel that here they do generate great nurses. I feel that they try new things and if it doesn't work, they are willing to go back to the way it was. I don't know why else it fits. I do like the people I work with, especially my own staff. I have my handful of those whom I don't like to work with. But for the most part, the staff I work with day-to-day are pleasant, and I enjoy working with them. Teamwork is a big thing, and I look at the team on my unit. I'm also looking at the team provided between three oncology units as well. I think it is something that we need to support each other, at the unit director level as well as at the staffing level. I think we do a good job of that, although it is difficult at times.

B: Are there any opportunities of any kind or atmosphere or values that are a good fit for you?

P: I'm not looking to go any further. I have considered it, but I'm not. Not for any reason here—it's just that my husband and I are so busy with our careers. My career is the more financial [lucrative] of the two of them. It has just been a nice place to work. It's not been extremely difficult but nothing stands out. I can't really think of anything. The people are easy to talk to and work with and they are available.

B: You were talking in general about how this organization really supports its people and that is one of the reasons you like to be here. Can you think of a specific instance when you got organizational support from someone when you were trying to do something?

P: From a staffing perspective, when I was significantly short staffed, they did give me some people who belonged to the float pool. I felt upper administration did assign people to me. I had at least two agency nurses assigned to me who were full-time as well as four nurses from the other oncology units. They stayed with me, initially it was going to be for three months, then two of them ended up staying with me full-time and two of them went back. I felt very supported at that time because had it not been for those six people, I would have been working everyday as a staff nurse and not using my skills as a manager.

B: They provided that backup. Now we have the fantasy questions. Imagine a roomful of new nurse managers, and you get to wish three things for them that would help them be successful in their new role. What would be your three wishes for them?

P: Adequate orientation. One of the things we did as a unit director group is to develop an orientation guide. It has all the resources in it. I did not have that as a new manager. I felt that if I had had this, it would have been much easier. And to know which of your peer group [can pull] strings in which areas. That is very important.

B: That's one wish—orientation that would include those aspects.

P: I have gone to many classes over the years in development. They were helpful, but I only took certain pieces back from them. There were enough pieces taken back that changed my practice on the unit for certain things. I didn't like being away from the unit for long periods of time, but I think they were very helpful in the first few years of being here. I would include that.

B: Your second wish is some sort of leadership training?

P: Yes. I think you need that.

B: What is in the leadership training?

P: HR things. I'm trying to think of some more. Gail Wolff, who does a lecture on "Queen Bee Leader," does one of my favorite lectures. I have heard it about three or four times during the course of my role. At first I thought it was ridiculous, but in the end when you start thinking about this lecture and how you control them [your staff], it really does make a difference on the unit. Talking to someone who has had very good experience, I don't want to be that person during the role-play, but I like to watch it, you learn a lot. I encourage my nurses to role-play. One of the scenarios is getting nurses to call physicians. I make them do this for the new nurses. They don't really like it, but I tell them to go through with their preceptor what they have to tell the doctor. That makes it more comfortable for them. I think role-playing in difficult situations.

B: Was the lecture on "Queen Bees"?

P: Yes, you always have nurses on your unit who are queens. Have you ever heard Gail Wolff speak?

B: No, I haven't.

P: You should. Initially I thought it was ridiculous but in the end I started thinking who played those roles on the unit in a negative way and how you can control them. Once it hit me, [I understood]; it took three or four years, but it did.

B: Then you realized she was right about that and then the role-playing came up. You did that in her class and other classes. That is part of leadership training; it's almost like behavioral rehearsal. That's two wishes. What is your third wish?

P: Learning how to orient new nurses. What is a successful orientation for nurses on your unit? Is it having that orientation guidebook? Or is it having them interact with the nurses you do have on the unit? To have a successful unit, you have to have a successful orientation. What happened to me was that multiple people had commitments and they worked for two years. At the end of the two years, they would all leave. I wondered why they were all leaving. I dreaded the six months before they left. I finally got through that, but I kept thinking, "How do you make orientation successful?" I have learned those things along the way.

B: I can see that is really central to success. That is something most of your colleagues are in agreement with. Each place does it differently. It makes a big difference on whether or not you come aboard in the end and whether you stay aboard.

P: I know I play a role in that and the staff plays a role in that. It's a combination.

B: In your mind, what is an ideal orientation?

P: The key is knowing what the expectations are. Knowing you have to get done by this date, and every week this has to be done. Having a guideline. I still don't have a guideline; I have a daily calendar. Knowing what organizational pattern is going to work for you. I have tried multiple patterns over the past five years, and the person who suggested this calendar to me gets the prize. I wouldn't use it for the longest time, but once I used it, it kept me in check. Just having that tool that is going to work for you. Having someone to make suggestions to you. Having some organization to your job each day.

B: Organizational skills would be an important part of that as well.

P: You do have to adapt them over the years. But having someone say, "This pattern works for me—it might work for you."

B: You would like leadership training that includes behavioral rehearsal, where to go for resources, organization aspects, HR aspects. Anything else?

P: Maybe how to deal with difficult physicians. I don't have a lot of difficult physicians—maybe just a couple of scenarios come up. I think dealing with physicians who are angry is very difficult to do.

B: It's interesting because I was actually going to say to you that physicians haven't come up in any of my conversations. I was going to ask you about that. You think that should be part of an orientation. What should the approach be in terms of dealing with physicians?

P: I think that is a good idea—I have not had any type of education in terms of dealing with physicians. I have been very fortunate in that most of the physicians I deal with are no problem. I have had maybe one or two whom I have had problems with. They are no longer here, by their choice.

B: Physician management would be part of that. Here is the last question: It is the year 2015 and there are no nurse manager vacancies, the tenure is an average of 10 years, and satisfaction is at the highest it has ever been. What would have happened to make this true?

P: For the nurse manager role, it would be finding that true balance between upper administration and yourself. Being able to meet their needs, but also being able to run that unit efficiently and from a budget perspective. If you ask staff nurses, ideally they want as many nurses as possible and based on the acuity. But if you talk to administration, you have to meet some guidelines. You need to find some way to flex the two together so you still meet the needs for both of them.

B: Anything else you can imagine that would have changed in the field or in organizations that would make the role less difficult?

P: For me, I think it would be ideal to have a free charge nurse on a regular basis.

B: How would that work?

P: Someone who would be rounding with your physicians but able to support your staff. Right now, I am the charge nurse on the unit. Having somebody there—if I'm off the floor for a meeting or anything, I can't support them. I would like to be able to support them more, and having the charge nurse would help. It's having the partner to work with, day in and day out. We have our clinician role, but 80% of the time they are in staffing. They are in staffing 100% of the time if you don't have enough staff. They can't support you in the way you need to be supported. I think as unit directors, we could really have people do much better in orientation, to support your orientees much better if you have this free charge nurse. I think that sometimes the staff do not feel supported when we are out for meetings. We need to be out for certain meetings. Again, balancing the two of them and having time it takes to do the job. There are many things you put off until tomorrow, and then tomorrow you put off to the next day. And it continues. I spent four hours over the weekend doing stuff I wanted to get done by Friday. I truly put in 12-hour days last week and then 14 hours on top of the last two because of the computer system being down.

B: Those are all of my questions. Do you have any questions for me?

P: No, I don't think so.

B: I wanted to know what it felt like to answer the questions for you?

P: Not as bad as I expected. When I look at my own personal interview skills, I don't think I interview well; I get tongue-tied easily. Sometimes trying to say what I want to say is hard.

B: Did you notice anything about yourself during this interview?

P: I think the resiliency. I don't think I really realized that not joining those people who were always negative has been beneficial. I knew it was, but I hadn't realized how important it really is.

B: When you are in charge of your own self, you can totally frame it how you want to. But there is that undertow when other people are doing it, and you avoid getting sucked into that. It's an energy conservation strategy as well.

P: If there is one thing I have always told my staff, it is [that if they would] just stop complaining and do the job, they would have the time and energy to do the job. They were very angry with me. I told them they were spending 20 minutes complaining being short staffed, whereas in 20 minutes you could be done with report.

B: You see that over and over again.

P: I think negativity really takes its toll.

B: It takes a lot of energy and thought process. That is a very clear strength that you have, and also your love for nursing really comes through as well as your capacity to sort of stand back and say, "I'm working on that." The way you talk about working on it shows that there is humility, but there is also optimism about it. That kind of ability to see yourself and how you affect other people is a really strong leadership skill that you have. It is interesting to talk to you. You do have a sort of "calm" and you are really settled. You have a positive core that is settled about loving this work and doing it and sort of figuring out whatever it is that you need to do. The core doesn't change. That is how it comes across to me. It is a key leadership strength. There is something about you that comes across as being very settled; it is beyond calm. I'm thinking it comes from your love of the work and caring for the patients. It comes out of your love for caring for the people who care for the people. What do you think?

P: I think so.

B: It's what you come back to. Having that settled core always sort of reels you back in. That is within you; I see it when we talk. You have that inner strength. You know what you have to do to get back to the place where you are responsive and not reactive. That is a real goal for you; that is how you wanted to remake the unit. I think it is also something you do yourself. . . . It is a pleasure to listen to you talk about your work and how much you love it.

Transcript of Full Interview

All identifiers have been removed to protect confidentiality. This six-year manager opens a window in her descriptions of how organizational and individual strengths can nourish and reinforce each other. Notice that she was nurtured by a significant and approachable mentor, in a culture of generativity and learning, and how she expresses her own brand of generativity. Keep your eye on her line of sight: She was attracted to the role because she could see how to use the management role to transform care at the bedside. She identifies with the work of her staff, counting her accomplishments in their development.

Use this interview transcript for your own research as a case study or as a discussion focus in class. As you read, try to identify the signature strengths of the individual nurse manager being interviewed as well as the strengths of her organization.

B = Interviewer

P = Participant

B: You have been six years in this role. I want you to go back to your beginnings as a middle manager here. Can you think back to anything in the beginning that seemed really promising or positive?

P: When I was first officially interviewed and offered the role, I had been functioning as a backup or assistant to my predecessor, so I had already been involved in some decision making and the mechanics of management. The thing I found most promising was that I was going to be in a position to help nurses get what they needed to take care of our patients. That was one of the big factors that was encouraging to me. I could really make a difference in the day-to-day functioning of a person who is really touching a patient and get them the tools they need and classes they need.

B: When you first got into the "meatiness" of your role, you could see that the role entailed giving people what they needed to enhance the care at the bedside. Do you remember any incidents back then, anyone who was particularly helpful, anything that went well for you?

P: My predecessor was promoted and she was still here in the building, so I think any questions I had, she was there to answer. Things that went well; it was an easy transition for me because I had some experience with "pinch hitting." I think the transition went well, in addition to me already knowing the staff there. I had worked side by side with them. There was already a trust between the staff members and myself. They knew my philosophy and expectations.

B: When you say "your philosophy," I know that to you that means a number of things. How would you characterize the philosophy that they knew about?

P: They knew that patients came first for me. The care that I had delivered was the same care that I would expect somebody to give to my family members. Although I know that everybody has a life outside of here, I have had trials and tribulations in my life outside of here and those were always left at the door to the best of my ability. So, whatever was going on peripherally, my patients always came first. I think I have always been a nurse advocate, even when I wasn't in a management role.

B: An advocate for nurses? What does that mean?

P: I have never been one to be afraid to express my opinion, whether that is to my detriment or not. I think the nursing staff that I work with, as well as management staff that I report to, knew that if they asked a question, they were going to get an honest answer. It might not always be the answer they were looking for, but they knew that would be my honest opinion.

B: You were straightforward. Can you tell me a little bit more about the person you replaced and how she helped you ease the transition?

P: We had a long-standing relationship because our first jobs as graduate nurses were working in a unit together. She recruited me from another health system hospital to come here. Nursing was not her first career; it was her second career. She was very education focused. She guided us all in that avenue. She was an advocate for nurses to promote the profession through education and experiences. Can you repeat the question?

B: The nature of her support for you. You talked about her being available if you had questions; how else did she support you?

P: In addition to being my manager and a co-worker, we had an underlying friendship. She truly was a mentor. When we talk about mentors, it doesn't necessarily have to be the person that you work with. Beyond our work relationship, she was someone who encouraged me outside of work, inside of work. She was sort of a cheerleader. Nurses, I think, historically are very bad at identifying their strengths or promoting themselves. She had a wonderful knack of pointing out your strengths as well as your weaknesses, but in a positive way—such as "If you want to achieve this, then this is what you need to do."

B: That would be a way of pointing out a weakness instead of saying, "You don't have any of this."

P: If you stumbled along the way, she would give you other ideas in a gentle way that you still felt support.

B: When you think back to her, what do you think you have taken away from that relationship that you use in your own leadership?

P: I think the encouragement. I have been very successful in the recruitment/ retention arena of the job. I don't know if that is because of our original manager. Maybe we modeled our own practice from that first GN position. She was very interactive with the staff, and I think the staff respected her because she could jump in and do their job. I think I have been able to model myself after that. People respect you if you are able to do what you are asking them to do.

B: Does that mean stepping in if someone is sick or actually just coming in and pitching in at the bedside?

P: It is a variation. I think when you hire new graduates, it is very easy to step in and take over. It is very difficult to mentor and guide people through that evolution of their practice. At times, yes, I would come in and staff if somebody was ill or if we had a hole in the schedule. [My predecessor] did the same. I think, more than that, the education process [was emphasized]. I focused a lot on the mentoring process.

B: In the style that she had? That sort of cheerleading and pointing out strengths?

P: Yes.

B: When you think back to that early time, are there any lessons that you learned from that time that you carry forward? We talked about one just now—the way [your predecessor] mentored you that was positive and supportive and very educational. Can you think of anything else from that early time that you learned that helped you succeed?

P: Early on, she identified one of her weaknesses, which is also one of my weaknesses. I think that I have grown over the years and she certainly has grown as well. The delegation piece of our role—it's very difficult for a person who is a hands-on person. If you start out with the practice of jumping in and being the hands-on person who will come in and fill the hole in the schedule as opposed to the person who will help [nurses] think differently about how to be successful through a day working short—that is one of the biggest things she taught me or started me down the road of better delegation.

B: Are you saying that something you learned was that she helped you reflect on the fact that you were like she was and then you were watching for it all the way down the line?

P: Yes.

B: Any other lessons? Not so much from her but just in general during that time that you thought were helpful and helped you succeed?

P: There are so many. The politics of health care. Sometimes learning when *not* to say something. That is very difficult for me. I continue to grow in that area. I don't think that I have given up my strong opinions; I am just able to continue to evolve the way that I approach sensitive matters in an administrative arena. I think that my approach with these staff members is still very straightforward with the selling of ideas: "Yes, I know this isn't something we would probably like to do or maybe agree with, but it's not to the detriment of patients so this is what we are expected to do, so we need to find a way to do it." Politicking.

B: Let's pick another card. Is it choosing your battles?

P: It is. That's one of her best lines. Pick your battles.

B: What are the other elements of how you would always hold strong opinions that wouldn't change, but if it's an administrative issue, you are choosing your battles? What else are you doing that is different in terms as more political?

P: I think the longer that you're in this type of role, you [begin to] see a bigger and bigger picture. You're not so "tunnel visioned" on "this is my area." You've grown from a staff nurse who is focused on your patient population, to maybe a charge nurse who is globally responsible for just your little area, to a manager who is responsible for the patients and the staff and the interactions with the ancillary services. I think the longer you're in there, [the more] you develop savvyness on which things are appropriate to [fight for], which things you might be successful at achieving or a positive outcome. Weighing the scales, is the battle really worth the outcome or is this something that really even matters in the big scheme of things?

B: That's what you've been honing. It's partly a big picture thinking in the end, as you were saying. Seeing it in the big picture helps you decide which way you really want to go and allow for it.

P: Correct, or maybe what's best. [For example,] in a very tunnel-visioned area, this might be good for the ICUs—that's wonderful, but it maybe would be negative outside of the ICU arena. So it would positively impact our area, but negatively impact other areas in the hospital and may be to the detriment of patients. That's not how we want it to turn out.

B: Yes—even seeing the biggest picture. Tell me one lesson learned during that time you said there were so many that you carried forward and have been helpful over the six years.

P: I have a trust in the practice of the nurses whom I work with. I don't know that my previous boss had such a trust in their professionalism outside of the patient care. Just the day-to-day functioning of the unit: giving people the power to control their schedules, letting them run council meetings, and developing people that way. Initially it's a huge leap to let go of that control, but you watch people blossom.

B: What moved you to the point where you were willing to do that? You said, "I have trouble with the delegation and giving away those pieces of it; that is a big deal."

P: I think that I reflected back on the original job that I had. The unit that we worked in was a very difficult unit but ran like a well-oiled machine. Our boss was one of those people who could jump in and take an assignment if need be. However, she also saw the value in developing other people. We had self-scheduling 15 years ago, and it worked so well in the high-functioning units. My goal for the unit I started to manage was that we would get over the reactivity-type mode and move to [being] a proactive group. Engaging [nurses] in those processes and making them responsible for their schedules and balancing the schedule—it truly helped them start to see a bigger picture.

B: You have a real capacity to sort of look around you and see what people are doing and take the lessons that seem positive and to translate them into your terms, but also see what's missing and do it a little differently.

P: I find that they didn't lack the ability, they just lacked the means. Nobody had empowered them to take control of this.

B: Yes, so you do it differently. Now tell me how you would explain how you have been here for six years. As you may not know, in the study the cutoff point to participate is five years or more in the nurse manager position. Some institutions have said that they don't have anybody that's been there for that long. You have been here for six years. How would you explain the positive factors that have influenced you to stay both in the role and in this place?

P: I've had the support that I desire in this role, [including] ongoing education. I think a big piece that a lot of organizations miss with middle management is that you are responsible for these enormous budgets and manpower and you're not really given the background [needed to take on these management tasks]. A basic nursing education does not give you the foundation to balance the budget or to manage people—I would even go as far to say [education on] appropriate communication styles [is lacking]. It gives you a basic foundation and most nurses just muddle their way through. [Institution name omitted] has the resources and the leadership at a higher level that sees or saw at that point in time that there were definite gaps and that picking a great clinical person and moving them to a management role, that's not always the wisest thing to do. One does not equate to the other, but [clinical and management skills] especially don't equate if you don't give [the new nurse managers] the tools that they need to perform the job. This place is very innovative and patient focused, so regardless if I had a management role or not, I was able to practice at the bedside and do new and innovative things. I think that is partly the reason why I stayed here in particular. In the management role, they have given me the tools that I need.

B: Just to look into that a little more closely, how did you get the tools? Did you take classes? Did you have coaching? What were the means of getting those things that you said are not part of a nursing education?

P: Actually, for all of those things, they send us to classes, leadership classes, within the institution. One of the first classes they sent us to was [run by] a chief nurse retention officer. That's what a manager is—so digging a little deeper into what makes people tick. You can't treat a nurse of 20 years and communicate with her the same way that you do a nurse of two years—so focusing on generation gaps.

They also sent us to DVI courses, which are also leadership. DVI is an international company . . . I think its original focus was business. Business—not necessarily nursing, but interview techniques, budget management, and those courses. In addition to formal classes, we've had coaching, not system-wide instruction, but the unit manager group as a whole would go to one of our conference rooms and pick apart our budgeting system. Not one-on-ones, but small-group activities.

B: How frequently would that be?

P: Monthly.

B: So you're saying that your perception is, I didn't learn the stuff I needed for this job in nursing school. One of the reasons that you have been able to stay in the job—and there are number of them that you talked about along the way—is you got the information that you needed and the coaching that you needed, like budgeting and interpersonal information, business information from a variety of coaching, cross-manager meetings, classes from people who came in from the outside to do it, and classes on the inside [of the institution]. You got a whole wealth of knowledge about how to do [the management function], so you felt that knowledge support for that information support.

P: Correct, there was information support as well as local experts. So even if you didn't really grasp the concept in your group instruction—for instance, in budgeting—we have a person who can pick apart a budget.

B: Like a go-to person?

P: Yes, we have a go-to person for just about every avenue.

B: Let's say that would be my weak point. I'm working on a budget and who do I go to? I can't figure out the budget. Who do I go to? Someone in nursing? Someone in the general hospital administration?

P: In nursing.

B: Is that their role? Or what role are they in? Or are they just known for being good at the budget?

P: Actually, that is one of their functions.

B: And what role are they in? Are they an administrator?

P: They are an administrator.

B: What is their job title?

P: Director of . . . I can't remember. You know titles change.

B: I was just interested to know that, because it comes up all across the country: People don't know who to go to for their budget. That's been resolved here. Is it by the force of personality or is she a designated person for whom budgeting is part of her job description?

P: That is part of her job description.

B: Can you think of any other factors that have influenced your decision to stay here for six years?

P: I think that after you have been in an institution for a five-year mark, you have a comfort level. You know the system; you know the go-to people. I think sometimes it's easier to stay than it would be to leave, unless you have some external motivating factor. There is a comfort zone.

B: It's interesting that I find myself thinking about the "five-year edge." This is the five-year stitch where you feel you are kind of tied in. You said earlier—I smiled because I knew, and so do you—that it is really hard for nurses to praise themselves and to designate things that they do well. So that's what this question is: What gifts, values, attitudes, and capabilities do you bring to the challenges of this role, and how have they allowed you to be successful?

P: I think it's the integrity, honesty, and trust. Those three things, I think, are in your upbringing just as an individual. They were something that was very important in my household growing up. A good work ethic. The "never tell a lie because you will be in more trouble for telling a lie than you would be for your actual offense."

B: Yes, I know government officials who do that.

P: Yes, I think those things [are important]. I think that I have good people and communication skills. We would go to classes in situational leadership, and I think that I do that well.

B: Tell me what each of those words mean to you: communication, people skills, situational leadership? If we were to do an anatomy of those, what would be the elements in them?

P: Well, I think they are all interlinked. I'm able to be a situational leader by evaluating a person whom I'm engaged with. I am able to adjust my communication style to what their learning or what their educational level is, or even as far as being able to detect their emotional [state], of where they are at that point.

B: You can read someone?

P: I read people well. And I think I'm a good listener. A huge part of that communication is listening to what the person is saying back to you or what they are not saying—so that's the reading the people part.

B: That's the reading people part. You know some people say listening [is the most important aspect of reading people], but to you it means a little bit of listening between the lines and what's not being said.

P: Yes—body language. I think that I am actually lucky that I worked with many of the people whom I manage so that I know a lot of other things that are going on, maybe outside of work or maybe inside of work. It's more at a personal level.

B: That's an advantage in terms of the strength [with which] you cultivated those kinds of relationships that have more depth.

P: It's an advantage and a disadvantage.

B: Is it a disadvantage because sometimes it's hard to draw a boundary when you know how difficult someone is?

P: It's very easy for things to become gray if you take into account everything else that is going on with the individual as opposed to just black-and-white policies.

B: That's really true, absolutely. So more of your strengths?

P: More of my strengths—I think I'm very education focused. It is important to me, and I think I'm able to guide people to see that this is an important part of the evolution of your practice. Maybe it's not a formal education. I have a lot of senior nurses who have no desire to go back to school, but I'm still able to engage them through informal instruction or classes here on campus. You continue to develop them in that arena. Every little bit of knowledge that they gain helps their practice and helps them, even if it's communication classes as opposed to some technical piece. I like to watch people develop. I think part of the reason that I like this job is that even with the senior nurses who have more years of experience, you still watch them grow.

B: And that's a strength, too. Not just to say, "Well, you have to grow because you will be good at your job," but it actually gives you pleasure; it's gratifying for you to see that. Anything else you want to add about yourself?

P: I don't think so.

B: What do you bring to the nurse manager role that allows you to connect with so many different people, because the cast of characters is pretty long? You mentioned some things that are really critical. You listen, you lead a person, and you recognize potential in people. What would you say in answer to that?

P: I think [you need to be] able to communicate with people by the listening piece—even patient families, to be able to judge the situation. I'm thinking maybe of a complaint situation, where a lot of times people just want to be heard. They really don't expect action, and they really don't expect a response. They just want to be heard. I think the "reading people" part is very critical. I think some folks who go into management positions maybe do it for the wrong reason. It's not about being the boss. Most of the time I will be introduced to a patient family by a nurse as "So this is my boss." I'm really just a nurse here; I just have extra paperwork to do. I think that's important—the communication piece and maybe being able to have a softer touch with people, not being afraid to touch a person or let them in your space. People need to know that you're a real person.

B: Those are all intriguing comments—a softer touch, not being afraid to touch people physically, and letting people into your territory or your space. Let me ask about having a softer touch: What does that mean?

P: People need to know that you're also a person, not just an administrator here in the building. Knowing that you care or having the perception that you care.

B: How do you get that across?

P: It's the listening thing. Engaging them in conversation and asking one or two follow-up questions in a conversation can sometimes lead you down a whole other path.

B: Right. It's that unchallenged presence when you're listening and going beyond. It's the follow-up that shows you're actually following.

P: Yes, yes. It's very easy to walk by somebody in the hall and say, "Hi, how are you doing," and you really never wait to get their response, you keep walking.

B: It is that real engagement.

P: Yes.

B: What does it mean to let people know that you are a real person? Just operationally, what does that look like?

P: Not positioning yourself behind a desk; getting out there, even if you do have somebody in the office area. I think I'm probably a lot different than other managers, because we have clinician positions here. For example, I've invited them all in. There are three desks in my office. I don't have *my* office—it's *our* office. I share my physical space. Not sitting behind the desk but sitting in a chair beside somebody can make all the difference. It's about taking down barriers.

B: That's part of what you mean about literally letting someone into your space. In terms of showing that you're a real person, is there an element of self-disclosure about your life outside of work with that or is it just a genuineness of response?

P: I think it's the genuineness. It's not always good to share your baggage. I think being able to engage people in conversations, and maybe sharing a little bit generically with them, [ensures] that they know that you do understand, without sharing specifics.

B: Yes, got you. Describe to me from your perspective what's satisfying and gratifying about your experience here in the nurse manager role. What gives you a sense of pride?

P: Watching other people grow and knowing that you are a part of that. Over the course of my tenure as a manager, we've grown my specific one unit from 14 beds to 22 beds, so there was a time where we had 17 or 20 new graduates all at one time. [I enjoyed] being able to be that supportive person not only to the new graduates, but to their preceptors, and watching someone evolve as an educator/preceptor/mentor to the brand-new person as well as watching those green people grow into a good solid practice.

B: In this setting, what does "preceptor" mean? It means something different everywhere.

P: In this setting, it would be a person who takes on a new graduate and mentors [that individual] through the whole orientation process as well as follows them for another six months.

B: Terrific—in addition to their jobs?

P: Right, in addition to their jobs.

B: Is it formal?

P: It is formal.

B: Okay, how much time do [the preceptors] spend with [their new-graduate partners]? Do they have set meetings?

P: For six or eight weeks, they are side by side.

B: Now let's go back to the part about you. You talked early on about how you have this mentor who was a cheerleader, and you could get into the role and see how you could enable people to do what they had to do. You then talked about the satisfaction of watching people grow. Eric Erickson calls that "generativity." I think it's a great word because you really are [linking] to a new generation. . . . Is there anything else that comes to mind when you think about what's so satisfying about this? Because your face just changed! You just went, "Umm," when I was talking about that.

P: I think that's the greatest satisfaction—watching new nurses grow. This job has enabled me to continue in my education and focus more in a management track, so my master's [degree] is going to be in administration, I'm able to gather more skills outside of the facility and bring them here and implement them. It's satisfying and gratifying to watch myself grow as well.

B: All at the same time. Lots of growth there.

P: It's all about growing.

B: It *is* all about growing. I want to ask you to describe for me now one experience, a standout and high point, one time when you just felt engaged, alive, just really in the flow, as they say. What made it such a memorable experience? Who was involved and what was happening?

P: I think probably one of the highest would have been when we successfully had all of those graduates off orientation, or a morning meeting when I said I have no staffing needs. Knowing that all of those people came out successfully: I hadn't lost anybody to board failures or anything like that; they were mentored successfully and functioning at a high capacity. [Knowing] that I played a part in making them successful or helping in their success.

B: And to look at them and realize that you are part of this work. If you take apart the aspects of how you participated, what would you say?

P: Beyond the organization of that number of people.

B: Yes, 17 [nurses] or something like that.

P: Between 17 and 20 [nurses]. Beyond the mechanics of getting those people through, I found it to be a personal success to be able to connect with all of those people and build relationships with them. Maybe I wasn't as close to them as I was to the people who I worked with side by side; those relationships are very different and are still different today. I think being able to engage them [was gratifying,] because you don't know them as well as you know the folks whom you've worked with for a long time. Being able to develop those relationships [meant] that there is a trust there, that they know they can still come to me, that I have an open-door policy and they will flood in.

B: It was a grounding of those relationships that started to develop.

P: I think that was one of my fears. All of these people—how was I going to engage them? And be able to pick apart what their driving force is, [because] everybody has different motivational factors.

B: Right. It's important for you to be able to figure that out, so that you can get [nurses] to work in the best way and keep them correct. So your most memorable time and what makes it gratifying are very much tied in together. What you find most gratifying is watching people grow, and that magic moment is when you look back and see that the new nurses are staying.

P: Yes, we've done it.

B: Yes, you did it. You said, "we." Who do you mean when you say that?

P: The whole team, at that point in time even up to the vice president level. I knew that this was a huge undertaking and that I couldn't do it alone. [The vice president] gave me permission to pull other people out of staffing to help follow them through orientation. I had the support of the VP as well as everybody on the unit.

B: That's interesting, because I had a question here about giving me an example of a time when senior leadership helped you succeed. That would certainly be one.

P: Yes.

B: You have the backup that you needed to really pull these people through.

P: Yes.

B: I want to have you talk about collaborating with the staff nurses. We were talking earlier about how you come in and do the job and sort of that balance. [Can you tell me] about a particular time when you collaborated with a nurse and it made a difference in the care of a patient?

P: Just in the past several months, one of the units that I have has a large oncology population. Very ill, sometimes young [patients.] It's usually not just one nurse—if you have a success, it's usually not just one nurse. They only work three days a week. A team of nurses was caring for a young man with children and a young wife, and he was with us for a very long time before he passed. I think that we had positive outcomes, maybe not with the patient himself—obviously he passed away—but we collaborated together, not only the nurses and I, but with our physicians, staff, and our palliative care staff, to be supportive to this young wife with young children. She has been in contact with us since, telling us what a wonderful experience she had and how supportive we were to her and what a wonderful leader I am. That's because of all these folks who work for me or for the house system. They are so compassionate and they are able to do their job because of the things that I let them do.

B: That's a wonderful, memorable time because you could see your people who have grown into the ability to be right to care for this family in a tall way.

P: And treat them like they would treat their own families.

B: Yes, you said that really early—that's the criterion. I meant to follow up with you about this, but even just remembering that story is so moving, isn't it?

P: It is.

B: It really takes you back. You mentioned the way that you were brought up, your family. Part of that brought into play [the notions of] integrity and sort of speaking your piece. Is there anything else about the way you were brought up that translates into your convictions or your MO or the way that you practice?

P: I was brought up in a very disciplined household. I am the oldest, so I was the experiment. I was very disciplined, but also very encouraged to take risks. You won't know unless you try, so I was never told, "You can't." "Why don't you" was sort of my mom's philosophy. My father was a disciplinarian and my mom was the encouragement.

B: How do you see that in yourself? How do you translate? Because you are a translator of what you observe, the models that you observe—so where did you go with that?

P: Well, my mom says I'm like my dad. I think I'm a blend of both of their styles. There is a time and a place for policy, procedure, discipline—those types of things. But there is also that softer side that I think that is my mom, the encouragement cheerleader.

B: Somehow you picked out the best of both of them.

P: Picked out the best of them and what I interpreted as the best.

B: Absolutely, that's what we do with those lessons. It's not dissimilar to what you did with your mentor—sort of observed her behavior and picked out what you wanted. I think you translate [those lessons] in your own terms. I want to re-ask you the question about a time when senior leadership helped you succeed, because it came up earlier in the discussion of the 17 orientees. Can you think of another time or ways in which senior administration or an administrator has helped you succeed? Is there another example that you wanted to put forward?

P: I have been fortunate to have or be in a position with the comfort level to ask for things that I think are important. People expect the truth and a reality from me. To achieve certain outcomes as far as infection rates and stuff like that, to achieve those goals, I have asked for specific supplies, specific resources, and a free nurse in charge without an assignment to achieve certain goals and data collection. And we had a severe decline, a drastic decline in infection rates. Because I was able to ask for resources, I was supported and achieved a really positive outcome for our patients.

B: We talked about your mentor that you had when you first came in here. Has there been another mentor along the way? Have you maintained the relationship with her?

P: No, that person is gone. She has moved on. I can't say that anybody has filled that role entirely but, like I said, there are go-to people for functional types of tasks. I don't know that there is a person who I view currently as "That's the kind of person I want to be or the kind of nurse or manager that I want to be."

B: It's interesting because when you talk about a mentor, it has a real element of someone that I would call an exemplar—someone that you want to look at where it isn't just being a cheerleader; it's also someone that you look to and get examples for leadership from.

P: Correct.

B: Let's talk a little about [institution name omitted]. How has this organization been a good fit in enhancing your success and longevity?

P: My focus has been good patient care, no matter what nursing role I functioned in. Even prior to being a licensed nurse, when I was a nursing assistant, that was my focus—good patient care. I think [this institution's] focus is that as well: high-quality interactive care involving all of the players. The players are the patients and the families, and [the goal is] engaging them in their own care. They are only with us for a very short period of time, and then they have to go do it on their own. I think that is part of the reason I have stayed here is the patient focus.

B: Anything else about this place?

P: When I interview people, whether they are experienced or inexperienced—I have worked in the academic setting for [name omitted] down the street as well as the community hospital setting, and I think [my institution] has a very unique blend of both of those worlds. It is very academic. We do very innovative things, and we have the resources and technical equipment type of things that the nurses really love. On the flip side of that, even in a 520-bed institution, we still have a community or family type of feel that we are able to carry through. You are not isolated to your one little unit. Even as a staff nurse, you know people in other areas.

B: That's what you mean by family, hospital-wide?

P: Yes, hospital-wide and floor-wide. For years, our VP knew everybody's name. How she managed that, I have no idea. She was a very dynamic person who had a gift for that. I'm not just talking nursing staff. She knew housekeepers' names and dietary staff's names. [The atmosphere] lent itself to that family type of environment.

B: That is something that is attractive to you as well. Anything else about this place that is a really good fit for you?

P: The focus on education, whether it is formal or informal. We have a wonderful administration that finds value and puts their money where their mouth is as far as providing educational support to me as well as to staff members, such as the advanced practice nurses—providing conferences and sending people to conferences. Not only is the institution patient focused, but it also lends itself to advancement of nursing practice.

B: In terms of education here, can you be specific about whether there is a nurse university here, continuing education, et cetera? Are there ongoing classes? What are the mechanics of the continuing education here?

P: We have system-level classes that every hospital can send their nurses or managers to. Some examples are HR type of classes, leadership classes, chief nurse retention officer classes, and budgeting classes. I think more of my focus is what we provide for staff nurses. A lot of institutions are very focused on the brand-new person and forget about the people who have been here for a long time. I think we still have the ability to engage those people.

B: You are very invested in how your people develop. It is important to you in getting the education. When you took a leadership class in-house, was it a class?

P: It was actually a series. Some of the topics were HR related, what you were allowed to say and what you were not allowed to say. Policy-based classes. Interviewing classes. EAP [employment assistance plan] classes. Nurse educators came and explained what things were being covered for our employees. We have classes on how to mentor or precept. There is something all the time.

B: Are they optional?

P: Some are optional and some are mandatory for a director. Some are not mandatory, but if they are scheduled on your unit director development day, then you should go.

B: Out of all of those classes you have taken all these years, what have been the most meaningful for you?

P: I really enjoyed the chief nurse retention officer class. I never viewed a management role as why people stay. I still only believe a portion of that. I believe that people do need to feel some type of bond with their manager. Even if they have a loyalty to patient care, if they don't feel supported by their management, they might leave. That class in itself sort of made a light go off.

B: Can you think of another time when you felt supported by your organization?

P: I think every new manager who takes on the unknown basically and is able to be successful in their job, whether that is reflected in their evaluation or tenure—I think to be successful in this job, you have to have some sort of support. As a new manager, being given those tools and being able to have the go-to people is a huge support and a huge driving factor [for success]. People's success [depends on] being given the tools they need. Not every institution is able to do that, whether because it is a resource problem or because there is a lack of attention to detail. You can't expect somebody to manage people or budgets without the appropriate education.

B: You get that here, though. I am really intrigued with this go-to person. If I am a nurse manager here, is it really clear who this person is?

P: Yes.

B: I just want to make sure I understand this part. This would be because of her job title?

P: Yes, her job title, as well as [the fact that] she is one of the people who teaches the budget class to us.

B: The other go-to people—how do you know who they are? Are you told this in a class? This is one of the biggest problems for nurse managers. They don't know who to go to with their questions.

P: We have good organizational structure, so if there are education needs, we have a director of nursing education. Denise is the education person and we know that. If there is a class out there to be had, she will know about it. Regulatory questions, we have Linda; we know that she is the regulator monitor person for not only here, but [another institution within the organizational group] as well.

B: So there is a real clarity about that, and that is a form of support, along with education, to back up what you think is a pretty good match for the challenges you think you are going to have?

P: Yes, it is very clear.

B: Now, it's time for the fantasy question. You have a room full of new nurse managers and you have three wishes for them as they move into this role. What would you wish for them?

P: Education, so that they have the tools that they need. The support of administration. With either of these things not there, I think you could flounder.

B: So a mentor who would provide what to them?

P: A mentor who would provide advice, plus emotional support for the first six months, and help them navigate through all the unwritten rules and hurdles that every person struggles through with every job. There are always the unwritten rules.

B: Yes, the unwritten rules. You don't find out what they are until you have broken one of them. So that kind of guidepost and education for whatever it is they need.

P: Yes, they need a toolbox.

B: If you were designing the toolbox, what would be in it?

P: Depending on what their background is, some people might be a novice as I was when they start their job. Communicating tools, interviewing tools, recruitment and retention tools, budgetary classes, and maybe a binder with all the go-to people in it.

B: I have been to places that have that. It is so critical to have that. Your last wish had to do with support. What does that look like?

P: An administrative portion of your organization that has a focus on nursing and that understands that although finance is important to any business's success, nurses need certain tools to provide good care. You need that supportive administration, not only of the nurse manager but also of the whole nursing practice.

B: The last question: Imagine you are on your way home today and you slip through a wrinkle in time. The year is 2015. All of the vacancies for nurse managers across the country are filled and the average tenure is 10 years. Nurse manager satisfaction is among the highest in the nursing field. What has happened to create this change?

P: They have a whole toolbox. They have the three things I talked about, my three wishes, as well as support on the bottom end as well as the top end. They have a go-to person or a mechanic person to help them with the daily tasks. The whole job can be overwhelming. It's not just patient care and it's not just finances; it's a multitude of things. You have the communication and all of the things you have to accomplish and do well but you still have the day-to-day evaluations, audits, et cetera. Somebody to help with all the paperwork.

B: Do you have a precedent for that here? Is anyone receiving that kind of help?

P: We do have business assistants, but I think [our institution] and the health system as a whole were in the process of involving the clinician role in an administrative track as well as an education track, so identifying future leaders and future educators. This is one of the beginning processes of that. I have been fortunate to have really good people in those roles and develop them in those areas. I guess I am in a better situation than other people. I have some of [people whom] I am mentoring into a management person.

B: So it's a little bit of succession planning? Is it formal at your organization?

P: Yes, it is succession planning and no, it is not formal here.

B: Was it your decision to do that?

P: Because of the size of my areas, my VP was very supportive in finding help. We don't have an assistant director position, so I was given leeway to have somebody to develop administratively. Historically, my clinicians on [unit name omitted] have been education focused. [We had] three educators and another person who moved on to another nurse manager role, so I mentored him to go that route. I have another one to mentor to that route. So it is informal in the health system and formal in my areas. Administration knows that those are my goals. I have a succession plan.

B: Well, this may inspire others if they see it as successful. I think it is going to turn out to be one of the keys in this area. It has come up in a number of my consultations and interviews with people, either how important it is or how they wish they had it.

P: As I reflect back to when I took this role, we did not even have clinician titles at that point in time, but that is sort of what my boss did at that point in time. You get to gamble before you actually have the responsibility.

B: It's a testing out on both sides. But it is also the beginning preparation. It's a grooming process. Those are all of my questions. I wanted to ask you how the interview felt. What did you end up thinking? How was it for you to answer the questions?

P: They are not difficult questions, but it felt difficult to reflect back and take apart relationships and how things evolved in your own practice. It was a good experience.

B: Do you have any reflections about yourself as you talk about your tenure here?

P: I have no regrets—that's the one thing. You would think over a course of six years you might have some misgivings. I really don't. I never had the intent early on in my nursing career ever to be a manager. But it has [turned out] well.

B: From my observation, you have a couple of threads that weave through everything. Your integrity and inner authority, mixed with an ability to look around you and take pieces that you can grow within yourself and strengthen your own leadership, but at the same time being delighted with the growth of other staff nurses and leaders as you are about your own growth. That is real commitment to keep growing your own mind and your own skill set, [just as you grow] the people around you. That has been so consistent in everything you said. You said you have to figure out what drives them, but I think that drives you and it moves you at the same time. That is a combination that shows intense commitment. It is just a pleasure to listen to that story unfold and be so consistent. I imagine you have heard that, too. It's a self-renewing, rejuvenating-type thing.

P: It's not unlike a bedside nurse, or at least in my own practice as a bedside nurse: Your successes are your patients' successes. Now your successes are your staff nurses' successes. Living vicariously.

B: It's interesting that you should say that. I'm looking for a word to describe it. I think it is so critical. What happens to a lot of nurse managers is that they miss the gratification that came with the direct care, unless they can have a feeling that they are still part of that direct care. You said this really early on, that you get for your staff the things they need to do their job; therefore, this is all part of it. Unless you can still see that you are caring for the patient, but in a different way, then you will lose the core purpose of why you are in this role. I am searching for a name of what this is. It seems to be so essential and it has come out repeatedly in conversations with your colleagues across the country. They all have different ways of putting it, but it all comes down to, "I'm still caring for the patient."

P: If you took this job because you didn't like that job, then that was the wrong reason.

B: Take that a little further—then what?

P: Because you really didn't care about the ultimate goal to begin with, which was the patient.

B: If you thought you were getting away from the care at the bedside, you are not.

P: No.

B: If you can't keep the connection that your core purpose is the care at the bedside, then this role is too hard to bear?

P: I would believe that. You become weighed down in tasks as opposed to a goal. You never achieve a goal because the paper keeps coming. There is never an end in sight. You have to have some type of accomplishment to rejuvenate.

B: For you, the accomplishment is your staff growing, but also seeing where the care goes?

P: Exactly.

B: We are looking for portraits of engagement, signature aspects of the institution, but also signature behaviors of nurse managers who are successful that are consistent. By the same token, each person to me, like you, is a rare gem, not like any other. For me, that is the fun and gratifying part. You and I have spent this time together and I have a sense of what you like out there and what matters to you and what your practice is. As much as I am looking for patterns, the joy is to see each person as a one-of-a-kind nurse manager.

Transcript of Full Interview

All identifiers have been removed to protect confidentiality. Underline the strengths of this nurse, who became a manager in the old neighborhood, the surgical unit where she "grew up." After 11 years as a manager, her examples telegraph her ardor about care at the bedside. She conveys attunement and gratitude toward her patients and the strengths of her staff. She leads by example with clear expectations and prizes her capacity to be direct and outspoken. Observe her reflective side as she draws upon the wisdom of her experiences.

Use this interview transcript for your own research as a case study or as a discussion focus in class. As you read, try to identify the signature strengths of the individual nurse manager being interviewed as well as the strengths of her organization.

B = Interviewer

P = Participant

B: Let's start with your beginning in this particular role as a nurse manager. How many years back?

P: Eleven.

B: Think back 11 years ago, to those early days, weeks, months. What was promising about that in the beginning?

P: What I liked about entertaining the idea of becoming the next manager on the unit was that I had worked on this unit a few years as a nurse, and I liked the idea of managing the same unit I grew up as a nurse on. Nursing is my second career, so I entered this unit on the ground running. I already had a bachelor's degree, but I worked as a nursing assistant because I thought it was important to learn from the grassroots up and to work with all levels of the nursing staff because I was not interested in nursing prior to this. I liked the idea of managing the group of people whom I had worked with because I knew them already, a good deal. I thought that would be beneficial for me.

B: The continuity, but what else seemed beneficial about staying with the game?

P: Well, I think because I liked the game—[that's] number one. I continued to like this type of patient population, so surgical patients are my forte. I already knew in my own mind what I thought worked and didn't work, so I thought I had somewhat of an advantage over somebody coming in from the outside because they didn't know how things worked. [I knew] maybe what I might want to change as the boss versus being the nurse on the unit. So I just thought it was an easy transition for me. Now other people will differ and say sometimes [hiring someone] new from the outside works better, but at that point in time I thought that I could add to and continue to build what had already been started. I thought that was a good thing.

B: So you liked the people, and you had the inside information, including ideas about how you might like to change it. That seemed like a good launch pad for you.

P: Yes, [it was] a comfort level fit. I need to feel comfortable where I am. I need to hang my hat on the same peg all the time—just like when I come into this room, I said I needed to sit where I would feel comfortable. It's not that I don't like change or I couldn't adapt to change, because God knows that in nursing you do that every single day, sometimes every single hour. But [there are always] things I can't control. [I want to] be comfortable with who I want to be, and so that was [a key consideration in taking the nurse manager position].

B: Do you remember anything else from that time that was positive as you took on the role? Clearly, there was a choice for you—and a good one, from all the things we've talked about. Can you remember anything from the early time that was good for the future?

P: I had been a manager in my other life, so I thought that I could bring some of what I had already learned and what I had failed at and what had been successful. I thought I had a little notch upward with that because I was a little bit older. I thought that would be more beneficial than bringing in a new nurse. I had some life experience outside of nursing. I not only had the comfort level with the patient population and the staff, but I knew the doctors. I appeared to be well liked by them, so I thought they would also be instrumental in helping me transition from a staff nurse to a manager of the unit at the time.

B: When you got into the role, which was comfortable and good from everything we've been discussing, do you remember anything happening that was really positive where you thought this is really going to work?

P: Maybe two things. I remember as I brought in a new staff nurse, everybody got their "aha" moment—that okay, this is going to work or I can do this now. I was walking down the hallway after three months as a new nurse now on my own and I thought, "I can do this; I can work this out." I had that same kind of feeling as a new manager as well. I think it was because the staff participated in the interview of who they wanted to manage that. I overwhelmingly was selected. That meant a couple of things, I thought: that I was somewhat liked and that they liked some of my ideas and some of my plan on moving the unit forward. I thought this was pretty encouraging.

And the other piece of that was my prior life was in dietary [work,] where I managed in a kitchen and I didn't deal necessarily with professionals. I dealt with a lot of transient people—mostly teenagers who were working after school, people on their stepping stone to college. It was [a group of] people who weren't really committed to the job for very long. It was very transient. In working with nursing, it was very evident that these are professional people—and I liked that. Not that I didn't like dealing with the teenagers, but it was a challenge every single day: Like on payday you knew nobody was coming to work, or you would tell somebody about the dress code three days in a row and they still didn't get it. It was just a whole lot of things going on with the teenage group at the time.

With professionals, you tell them and by and large they mostly listen, and I like that. Not only do you tell them, but you get a lot of great ideas from them, and you are no longer the expert in everything. I surround myself with the experts. I am not intimidated by that—I like that, and I just felt further challenged because of that.

The two moments were one day I was walking down the hallway and I thought, when staff would come to me and say, "This is broken and this is what we would like to do to fix it," and I would say, "This is pretty good." I no longer had to have all the answers; I just needed to build the team that would have the answers and solve the problem. And then the other piece of it was that dealing with professionals at large was a lot nicer than dealing with a group who were not as committed or transient because of a million different reasons.

B: You could see the potential there in how much further you could manage them, if they were all committed professionals. When you think back to that time and its promising start—like the way you were elected, the vote of confidence—you realized you wanted to be there, liked the people, liked the work, the particular patient population, the unit at that time. If you think back to that time, and you think about lessons carried forward from that time that helped you succeed over the 11 years of being in that role, what would you say these lessons were from that early time?

P: I don't know if all the lessons are exactly positive. This is hard work; it is not easy being a middle manager. You feel it from all sides. This hasn't been easy, but I want to give credit to the people I work with, because the nursing leadership here the entire time I've been here has been very progressive and very hands-on and very patient-focused and also very bedside nurse-focused. I also have attributed a lot [of my success] to my own personal religious background and my family values and my work ethic and all the great things my parents did in raising me. I think that plays a great deal [in my ability] to handle this very challenging job every day.

B: I want to move what you just said to the next question, where we talk about your strengths. What you told me just now is that a lot of your ability to deal with this role comes from spiritual practice and ideas and from the way that you were raised. Let me ask you about lessons that you learned on the job in those early days when you were first nurse manager, and how you have kept with those. Apart from what you have learned at home and your religious practice, what was the actual learning you had as a staff nurse [that contributed to what] you are now as nursing manager? What did you learn that really stayed with you?

P: Well, I can't really separate [that component out] because who I am and what I am are because of how I was raised and what I believe. But a part of the lessons learned is "Follow the rules." That keeps me honest, and that is one of the things that I have really tried to do over the years. As I gain more scope of responsibility, [I have tried] to follow the rules and not deviate from that because that keeps me fair across the board for everyone. Whether it's patient fairness, employee fairness, or whatever—not that it doesn't mean I don't make exception to things, but by and large I follow the rules, so that people know where I'm coming from.

The other piece of it is from past bosses whom I have had. It has been very important for me to always know what is expected of me and how I can be successful in my role, whether I was working as a dietary [staff member, a nurse,] or a student in college. I try to give that back to my staff. I try to let them know what the expectations are from the get-go. And I try to keep a very open forum if they have an issue or concern, a good thing, a bad thing, a positive or a negative, or whatever. I have an open door for that, and I have time for that.

I see them later doing the same, whether while precepting new nurses or new staff or in how they handle different situations. It's kind of leading by example. So it's following the rules, leading by example, treating others how I would want to be treated—that is so important to me. Taking care of patients when they are sick is really difficult, because they are not always themselves. You are not at your best moment when you're sick or when you have just received really bad news or when you thought they were going to take one piece of an organ out and they ended up taking all of the organ out. That is frustrating. You deal with a lot of things emotionally, physically, technically. It's hard. I think it's important to be that sounding board for the staff—to be available, to be able to have them say, "Hey, I'm having a really lousy day today," and you can figure out things. I tell the staff, "I don't ever want you to go home crying in your car. If you do, then we need to talk about that and we need to figure it out. Or if there was a really difficult patient for you, we need to make sure you don't have that same patient 10 days in a row, because you don't need that." Just because our job can be difficult, it doesn't have to be hard every single day, and I try to portray that to the staff.

B: You're talking about the values and standards that you lived by as a nurse manager, and you said that these were sourced in your religious upbringing and in the way your parents brought you up. Can you talk a little more in particular of the values, attitudes, and capabilities that you bring? What attributes and skills are those?

P: I am very organized. The newer managers, anytime they are looking for a hard copy of anything, they call me; they know I have it. So I am kind of the joke of everyone. And it's the hard copy because I don't trust the computer. So I would say being organized has helped me a great deal.

I'd also say being able to laugh at myself, because you can't take everything so seriously. I'll do something really stupid, and I'll be able to sit back and laugh. I think that people then see you're a little bit human, and that's important.

I always thank people. I try to pat them on the back—even though they say don't even touch people anymore, I still pat them. I guess it is part of my Italian background. We talk with our hands and we're very "huggie" types. I will pat someone on the back and say, "How are you today?" or I'll try to remember something small about everyone, like they got a new dog or they bought a new house or maybe they told me they had a death in their family. I try to do something individual so people don't think that I'm at large addressing the group, but I can be very individual. I try to do that.

B: Important information about making it a point to remember and make the connection to them.

P: When I go away on vacation, there is a particular person who always fills in for me. She'll say to me, "I just wish you could leave your brain here, too, because I don't know how you keep it all in your mind. You know exactly where everything is and where everyone's at and what everyone is doing, and you don't have it written anywhere." That's part of coming from a large family; you have to learn those things because you want to just survive. So I think that's another thing that I'm pretty lucky at remembering pockets of things.

B: On one end, you got the hard copy, and on the other end, you got a really good memory for details—including personal details, what is going on with everybody else. You look at the fact that some of this training came from being in a large family. How large?

P: There were actually ten of us, but there are only six living. My father died very young as well, so we all had to kind of survive. Everybody did their little way of surviving, and mine was getting very organized and learning to be confident. I remember when my father died, he was the Italian father that took care of the family, but now he was gone and here was my mom, who didn't even know how to write a check. I thought, "I will never, ever be like that." That was just the driving force behind me to take charge.

B: To take charge—and part of taking charge is being organized, knowing where everything is. You sound like you have a really amazing mental retrieval system, mental filing system, and physical paper filing system. Anything else about yourself that you bring that allowed you to be successful and work long term?

P: Well, I have a big mouth.

B: What do you mean by that?

P: I just put things out there rather than just talk about someone behind their back or be angry and never have it resolved. Life is too short and there is too much to do; I don't have time to waste in my brain on those kinds of things. I will be the one often in a group who will raise my hand and say, "You know what, I'm not comfortable with that." I have learned over the years to be much more eloquent and state things. I used to sit there and people would say my expressions were all over my face. I have learned to [manage] that much better. But I still put things out there, though, because I think it's important. Nurses have [sent the message] for so long that "We can just fix everything. Just keep giving us the dirt and we'll just keep shoveling and put our boots on and go right though it." Yet you look at all these other professions, and they won't tolerate that. Why does the nurse always keep doing more? When you think about it in terms of just salaries alone, there were people who were picking up garbage who were making more than a nurse who was saving somebody's life. And we just sat back and let it happen to us. I didn't understand that. I didn't understand because I joined the profession later and I wasn't just going to sit there and take it.

B: You said, "big mouth," but that has the connotation when you describe what you mean that you are direct and are outspoken.

P: Yes.

B: Why are you laughing?

P: Because that's exactly what people would say about me: I am direct and outspoken, although not much laughter.

B: How do you make that work for you?

P: Right, because you look like the complainer and that's not what it's about. I have learned to rephrase things. You do get what you want when you get good at that. That just took years and years of doing it. And practice, a lot of practice—when you manage people, you practice a lot. The first negative time you have somebody in the office because they didn't do something right, that is really uncomfortable. Maybe you don't do it very well and that person leaves feeling inadequate, and that's not what you meant to happen. The more you practice it and the more you talk and the more you say, [the better you get at communication.] And be honest: I'll say, "This an uncomfortable discussion we are going to have. You may not like a lot of the things that I need to say, but it's important that they are said and these are the reasons why." We are here for our patients, and you get better at it because you practice. I have had ten years of practice, so I hope I'm better today than I was ten years ago—but I am open to that and to learn to do better.

B: It's an art form, in terms of expressing an opinion that might be a little bit against the tide, but that you feel you have to speak out about it. Anything else you want to add in on that particular question?

P: No, I don't think so.

B: Okay, I want to skip back. You have been [in the nurse manager position at this institution] for 11 years. How would you explain the positive factors that have influenced your decision to stay in this place, in this job?

P: A couple of the things. The very reason I took the job was the patient population. I continued to want to manage patients who are surgical [patients], because that's what I like. Also the other thing that hit right on from the beginning of this job, and continues to do so today, is that the confidence and the skill of these nurses are phenomenal. They are so good. Doctors fight to get their patients on my floor because of the skills that these nurses have. It overwhelms me; I feel so honored to work with such a gifted group of people, and that continues to be the driving force [behind my longevity]. If I had a bunch of people whom I couldn't respect confidence-wise, there would be no way I could do this, because it's difficult and it's hard. But [I know] when I'm not there, they do cartwheels over anything that needs to be done. This continually happens time and time again. I was just on vacation last week. I came back today and at least ten different people said, "Your group was just phenomenal last week." It constantly wows me about their skills.

B: What do you think and feel when you hear that, "Your group is swell?" What do you think?

P: I am satisfied, I'm appreciative, I'm overwhelmed, I feel so fortunate—all of those things, because it's amazing what they do.

B: You said in the very beginning that one of the real attractions was the professionalism of the people with whom you work. Now we add to that the confidence and the autonomy [you enjoy] because they are being able to function and keep things running whether you're there or not. Any other positive factors for you that would explain why you are able to stay in the role?

P: Well, I can't say it's the hours, and I can't say it's the workload. Some days I ask myself, "Why don't I just work three 12-hour shifts like everybody else?" But I like being the boss. I like being in a position where I can be in charge. I like to be a change agent, not only in today's decisions but in tomorrow's policy as well. I think I better serve nursing at large doing what I'm doing than being the bedside nurse. But who knows? I feel so fortunate that tomorrow I can make the decision to go back to the bedside and it would still be a win-win [situation] for me. I feel lucky, and not everybody has that opportunity. Now I know I can go all over the country and work because of the nurse shortage, and basically write my own ticket. A lot of people worry their entire professional life about job security and job confidence and will this company be here tomorrow. There is always going to be a need for nurses. Because I don't have to worry about that, I can concentrate on so many other things that will make a difference. Does that make sense?

B: Yes, that part is probably true about nursing in general. I am interested in what you said: "I can write my ticket so I can go someplace else, I can be a staff nurse, and I can always go back to the bedside." My question is, What keeps you here? You said your colleagues, your staff nurses, keep you here. What are some other reasons why you wouldn't say, "I should write my ticket someplace else"?

P: Because of the nursing leadership at large here, the executive level of leadership. It continues to challenge you, it continues to listen to you, and it provides opportunity. We just received our letter that our Magnet application went through. We are in our phases of getting together for that, and we are very involved on a national level, as a Transforming Care at the Bedside (TCAB) unit, and with Robert Wood Johnson [Foundation] and IHI [Institute for Healthcare Improvement]—it's not just this little hospital in this little city in this state. It's phenomenal. In the last ten years I have traveled as far as Finland to go to an international nurses symposium. Two weeks ago, [I was] in Boston; this fall, I'm going to Denver and Miami. It's amazing. I was in San Diego a few years back. I never thought in nursing you would travel if you weren't a traveling nurse. And yet I am getting this opportunity to learn from the best in the country and to be a part of it and to hear [this hospital] announced [as a model] at these national conferences because of what it is doing at the bedside for nursing. It's fabulous.

B: So part of that is just the identification with this growing positive profile of the place. You also said that your senior leadership gave you opportunities and challenges. Tell me a little bit about that. Is that what you meant about the meetings?

P: It's all of that. Very much like when I say to my staff, "This is the problem, this is the problem, this is the problem." Then I say, "Okay, what do you want to do?" When they first started coming to me with "This is a problem, this is a problem, this is a problem," they expected me to fix it. Now they come in and say, "This is the problem and this is what we want to do." They don't even let me say, "What do you want to do?" They already know what's going to come next.

   Our nursing leadership is the same way. You don't come to the table and say, "I have a problem with that;" you have at least three ideas on how you want to fix that problem. What's really neat is usually—more times than not—they will listen to you. The VP and the nurse executive group will listen to some of your ideas and often may adopt them or trial them. We test [the new ideas] and do different things. That is part of the nursing culture here—that you just don't say, "This is the problem," without coming up with an idea. That's what I mean about challenge—that your thinking is stimulated constantly.

B: To think strategically is part of the culture. Is there any sense of where that came from or has it always been like that for you? It seems to suit you well.

P: It's always been like that for me. I don't know how far back that started to be created, but a lot of it was founded with Bill Wolff, who's nationally known as a nurse leader and who was the VP when I started. . . . It's been inherited in the bloodline, if you will, of the hospital. It's the DNA [of our institution] that we continue to cultivate this type of thinking and stimulate this kind of thinking.

B: And stimulating.

P: It is very stimulating.

B: From what you said, it's kind of your natural style anyway to just jump in and solve it. All these reasons [prompt you to stay,] even though you could write your own ticket, you could always go back to staff nursing and come up with a whole "writing other plans" script. It's that you're where you want to be right now, because of all the reasons that we talked about.

P: And I like the comfort. I only live 2.5 miles from here, so that is a huge win for me. Yes, my days are long but sometimes I am already at home, sitting down for dinner, while some of my staff who are going to [another county] aren't even there yet. It's that give and take. I don't feel bad staying here a little bit longer because I'll be home real quick. I need to hang my hat in the same place for a long time. I still live in the house I was born in. I need that safe zone and I have that here.

B: You know what it is. Did everybody else move out?

P: Yes, everyone is gone. It's just me and my mother and my two dogs.

B: I'm thinking now about this cast of characters, with your senior leadership, with your staff, your colleagues, patients, and families. What do you bring to this role that allows you to keep in step with all different kinds of people and all different kind of roles?

P: Well, it probably sounds like a cliché, but it's all about the patient. I will tell the staff that if you are not happy here, please leave. Do us all a favor, but most important do the patient a favor, because if you're not happy here, you are not giving good care. Patients aren't going to be satisfied. Co-workers don't want to work around someone who is miserable, and you don't want to be here when someone is miserable, so go be happy. I mean that in the most genuine sense of the word. All my decisions are based on the patient, because that is why we are here. For those who don't believe that, you can see that they are not happy with their jobs, and maybe not happy with life in general. Again, that keeps me very focused. [My] very "follow the rule" mentality [helps, too.]

It's all about the patient, and we have to figure it out if the patient is unhappy and why. Or we have to figure out what we could have done different in this patient's continuum of care. There is always a choice; it may not always be the choice we want, but there is always a choice. That's probably the number one thing: It's all about the patient. Not all the patients are crazy, and not all patients don't know what they are talking about. We have very, very informed patients today. Often they know sometimes more than we know, because they have time to sit with their computer and figure it all out and we don't. So I continue to drive that force—that it's the patient, it's the person in the bed.

B: How does that allow you to make working analysis? What you are talking about in a sense is an idea that connects you to anyone you might be dealing with: The patient comes first. But what qualities or abilities or style do you have that allows you to deal with so many different people throughout the day?

P: You mean, what I do personally to make that happen? I try to remember or pull a personal reach to my staff members; I try to do that with whomever I am interacting with—whether it's a patient or physician or ancillary department or whatever. Sometimes people just need to see it differently or explain it differently, so sometimes I'll try to do that.

An example is I have this gentleman who works night shift; he is a nursing assistant, thinking about nursing school. This was a change of career for him. I think he kind of worked in factory-type work. He dealt with machines and inanimate objects, and now he is dealing with people. He is a little rough around the edges. On four occasions in the last four months, about once a month, a different patient complained that he seemed a little rough, or he wasn't really listening to what they were asking; he was telling them what he thought they needed. We had to pull him in the office. I told him, "We have to talk about this." First you hear one patient say it—it could have been that the patient didn't feel good, or [the nurse] may have answered something inappropriately. You don't really hit the panic button, because for that one patient who may be complaining there are 100 patients who would say you are doing a great job. I try to weigh that as well, but this was the fourth time now.

So we called him and said, "What is happening here?" He was so upset that we blindsided him and didn't give him any heads-up on what we were going to talk about. It was kind of hard to give him a heads-up because he works nights. When we came in the morning, we said, "Do you have a minute? We want to talk to you." He said, "I am very angry and upset." We let him talk to me and to the clinician who works with him. We let him talk and voice his opinion.

Then I said, "Your opinions are important and valued, but I do need to tell you that this is what this patient said—and this patient, and this patient. What I am seeing is a pattern here, and we need to figure out what are we going to do about this pattern." I said to him, "You were angry and upset and blind-sided; so was I when this patient called me into the room and said that you know your employee is doing this, this, and that."

I said, "Do you not think I was blind-sided by your behavior, that I was now getting yelled at because of what you did? How do you think that made me feel?" And he looked at me and said, "I never thought of it like that."

I said, "It's not about you and it's not about me; it's about the patient. But I told you that because you have to understand that a patient in a bed is vulnerable. [When patients] ask for a pain pill, watching that clock seems like hours, when sometimes it's only minutes because they are in pain or they are afraid or they are uncomfortable or they are angry or whatever. We need to follow through on things."

It's just important that I tied it all into the patient and to the patient experience. But it's okay doing that: The staff have a good experience, and they walk away with something positive as well. It's not all punitive; it's not all not considering what the staff feels as well. I don't want it to sound like I make every decision based on the patient without anyone else's input, because that's not really the case. It kind of all happens together.

B: We were talking about how you connect with so many people and giving feedback to that particular person. I didn't get to the end of that sequence for you. Was the way that you dealt with him an example that is pretty typical for you in terms of how you deal with people?

P: I try not to make it personal. I try to make it whatever the subject is, number one. I'll tell staff, "You are not bad people. You may have made a bad decision, but that does not make you a bad person." Doing that takes away some of the harshness but still drives home what you are trying to get at, or [helps you] to make your point. Even when I talk with physicians, if I try to really pose [the question]—and often I do—as something like "Ms. Smith in this room is having this difficult time with me," not as "because I want you to make my job easier." I take away that personal piece of it and try to put out the facts of the subject. That seems to work because people get defensive sometimes. I don't want to do that, because that has been done to me and I don't like it. I am uncomfortable with that [blaming approach.] I try not to let things that have happened to me in my life that I think weren't really good experiences—I try not to re-create those same scenarios with somebody else.

B: You learned that somewhere. In the case of the nursing assistant whom you were talking about, how were you able to make the facts for him, because it sounds like he got really upset about being blindsided and you said, "I feel that way." How did he end up feeling at the end of day?

P: He still continued to disagree [by insisting that] patients are sometimes crazy and that I really shouldn't listen to them. I said, "You know what, that is really not the case. I don't disagree that some patients may have some psych issues going on, but we still need to figure out how we can best care for a particular patient and [his or her] nuances, and not just think everybody is crazy so therefore you can say whatever you want to. That is not how it works here." I think he got the message, but I think part of that was some of the factory mentality that he came with.

B: Well, you had that in mind. Did you see a change?

P: We only just talked with him, not even a week ago, so we will wait and see. Also when we talked to him, we said, "You know, if we were giving you your evaluation next week, this would not be the focus of your evaluation; this would be a piece of your evaluation. So if we had a pie of ten pieces, this would be one-tenth of one of the things we were talking about. We don't want you to walk away with thinking you are no longer doing a good job. You have an area that you need to work on, and that's what this is about."

B: Okay, I want to turn now and ask you a different question: What is satisfying and gratifying about your experience in middle management and what do you contribute that gives you a feeling of pride?

P: The people I work with are what really gives me the greatest feeling of pride. There are countless patient stories that are just phenomenal. If I sit and think about it, I often cry, because it's amazing how we deal with the surgical oncology population, who are often our age. I'll walk past the room and I'll see a nurse just sitting there, holding a patient's hand and just talking—asking her, "Go ahead and tell me about how you are feeling. What does it mean, when you say you are going to call your husband and tell him that you are dying?" It's just amazing. It's amazing because even with all the technology, all the medicines, all the procedures, it still comes down to sitting at that bedside holding someone's hand when they are in their lowest moment. I see that on a daily basis. Or [I might] get a "thank you" note from [the family of] a patient who has passed away, saying what a difference the staff made in the last three weeks of their life. It's amazing. We have a quilt one patient made while she was dying; the day before she died, she finished it and sent it to us. Those kinds of stories.

I can go on and on because that happens all the time, and it's because of the people I work with, it's what they do. They do it so well; they are amazing, amazing group of people. When people talk about my units, I am overwhelmed with pride for that, because they do a really good job.

B: You identify with that and feel pride and a part of building that. The next question is related to some of what you just talked about. I wanted you to pick out one experience that was a real high point for you.

P: I just nominated the entire staff for an Ace Award for this one. It was a Friday afternoon and I was sitting in my office. It was about five o'clock and I was getting ready to call it a week, when I heard this uncontrollable sobbing. My office is at the end of the unit and there are two public restrooms there, so I really thought it might be coming from the public restroom. I don't panic all the time; sometimes people just need to cry.

The crying wasn't stopping, so I went out and both of the restrooms were empty. I went around the corner around my staff lounges. When I went in there, [I saw] two nurses, a woman probably in her fifties, and another woman about 26 with an infant. The woman with the infant was holding the infant, staring a blank stare. The other woman, I later found out, was the patient's mom. The patient was the husband of the woman holding the baby. The mom was hysterical; she couldn't even catch her breath, she was sobbing so uncontrollably.

I went in and said, "What happened?" One nurse said to me, "The oncologist was just in and told them that [the patient] had weeks to live." Now the patient doesn't know this yet, the mother is hysterical, and the wife is just sitting there. The one nurse looked at me and said, "She is going to pass out. We need to do something with her." So I said, "Call ED and see if there is someone who can see her right away and give her something." The wife said, "I just need to get out of here," so another nurse said, "I will take her down to the courtyard." A third nurse was in the room with the husband. All he knew was that his mother was hysterical, his wife was just staring, and he didn't know anything that was going on. So [the nurse] was in there [with the patient].

I called pastoral care and let's get the doctor on the phone and find out what he said, because we don't know if this patient has anything. So we get someone to talk to the patient, who was only about 28 himself. Everybody was just taking care of something. With the nurse who took the mother downstairs, the mother said, "I don't have any formula for my baby." The nurse called her husband and told him to go to [the grocery store], buy formula, and bring it to the hospital—and they did that. Pastoral care, when I went down to the nurse's station to get a hold of them, had already been called by the secretary at the desk. Everybody was just taking care of everything; it was just amazing. It was unbelievable how they handled this whole situation. Then we got the doctor back on the phone, who came up. We went into the room and we talked to the patient. It was just amazing in seeing that well-oiled machine [the staff members] doing something that they do every single day, but with such dignity and such respect for the patients. Even the ones who weren't actively involved were out taking care of everybody else's patients. You would never have known that a crisis was occurring on a Friday at 5:00 when usually all your support systems are gone, pastoral care is out of the building, and social work is out of the building. It was a Friday afternoon—it was amazing.

That was just a few months ago, but there are a hundred stories.

B: Again, looking at the people that you supervise what they are able to do—they go way beyond the call [and work] so wisely and so collaboratively.

P: And then there are those [interventions] that I've seen—how many interventions that a nurse has done and saved someone's life from a very technical point, by knowing what to do and the right things to do. I don't want to say it's all about hand holding, because that's not the case, either. A nurse may get so good with her skills. You can walk in the room and just know, "This patient is going" or "I've taken care of this woman four days in a row and she just doesn't look good and something is going to go wrong."

B: What comes through again and again is this common thread of just the pride you have about some of the people you work with and what they are able to do. I want to ask you further questions on that point, about collaborating with staff nurses on the care of the patient. Has there ever been a time when you partnered with a nurse who made a difference in the care of the patient? Where you directly came in and partnered with them?

P: As good as my staff are—and they are very good—and as confident and comfortable as they are, by and large there are some who just don't feel very good when interacting with the physician, if they feel that a physician is going one way and the patient wants to go another way. We often have this scenario [come up] because some of our surgical oncologists are doing some pretty innovative interventions. They may be one out of five surgeons in the country who are doing this [particular treatment]. So we get a lot of people [patients] from out of town. We get a lot of people [patients] who have had their one, two, three, or four surgeries and now this is the last chance—and this is just palliative and it's not for cure. Sometimes a patient will come and say to the nurse, "I don't want any more; I'm done." Then you will have the surgeon who is being very aggressive.

We had one surgeon about two months ago who ordered this biopsy of the liver where the patient said, "I'm dying; I don't want any more." The patient couldn't say that to the surgeon, but felt very comfortable saying it to the nurse. The nurse validated it. The nurse asked, "Do you not want me to intervene here?" and [the patient said], "Yes, I do."

The nurse came out to me and said, "What are we going to do? This is what the doctor wants to do; this is what the patient wants to do; the family really wants to do what the doctor wants to do. But I'm the patient's advocate. What do you think we should do?" I said, "Let me go talk to the patient." Again the patient validated that "I'm done; I don't want anything." I said, "We need to tell the doctor that." [The patient] said, "I just can't." I said, "You need to—it's your body and your decision. It's not like you haven't tried and didn't go along with it all along to this point, but it's okay to say you are afraid. It's okay to say, 'I don't want any more.' That's really okay."

I think that was all she really needed to hear. It's not that the nurse didn't say that, but I think she just didn't feel confident of going against the doctor. We are an acute care hospital, where you are supposed to try to do everything you can—but sometimes people don't want to do it. They want to be able to say, "I'm done," and they want other people to say, "It's okay to say that."

B: And you are joining with your staff nurse and validating that. You were able to put it to the fact that it was the wishes of the patient?

P: What was so amazing was the one surgeon was not going to do any more, but the other one—who was rounding because he was in the operating room and they had not connected yet—ordered the next test to have the liver biopsy. They already knew that they were going to do that anyway, and not do any more, but the surgeon hadn't connected with his partner yet. It really was the right decision.

B: As it turned out, you helped her put her wishes into effect.

P: I think she just wanted it validated, and then my nurse wanted to validate it. It was okay to say, "No, we are not going to send her down for this liver biopsy." They asked, "Are you okay with that?" and I said, "Yes, I'm more than okay with that. We don't make anybody do something they don't want to do."

B: Okay, now a completely different subject—your interactions with the administrators and senior leadership. You've talked about how senior leadership challenges you and that [the institution has a] sort of culture of "What are your ideas for fixing this?" Can you give me a specific example of a time when an administrator or manager helped you succeed or how this administration or managers have helped you succeed?

P: About four years ago, we really saw the leadership, in my opinion, step up to the plate for our staff. That had to do with our hours per patient-day—the patient acuity system that we have. Each unit has a number that translates into how you staff the unit per shift, with nurses, nursing assistants, et cetera. Prior to four years ago, we were a surgical floor, but it wasn't all surgical oncology. We would do gallbladders and hernia repairs and bypasses and things that we call simple surgeries. [When the oncological staff was brought] over here, they wanted a floor designated for surgical oncology patients. That's your liver, your pancreas, your colon, your stomach, and all the big tumor resections that go on—where the patients are really acutely ill for a number of reasons.

A lot of them already had two or three surgeries; a lot of them are debilitated from chemo and radiation. The more surgeries you have, every time [the surgeons] go in, you have adhesion, you have complications. And then we deal with some of these procedures where they put the chemotherapy agents right in the guts. Not only does that kill local light cells, but it also kills good cells—there are a lot of wounds and drains and tubes. The acuity is phenomenal. From taking care of our simple gallbladders and simple colon resections, [our unit] turned into this massive [caretaking of] surgical oncology patients. It wasn't just five or ten patients; it was 80% of my patient population, so at any time 30 of my beds are filled with these types of patients.

B: High maintenance.

P: It is; it requires a lot. It requires a lot of blood products; it requires a lot of potassium and magnesium supplements on top of NG [nasogastric] tubes, Foleys [catheters], films, and tons of different things. The acuity really went through the roof—but we weren't staffed for the acuity to go through the roof. We were allowed to have five nurses on day [shift], five nurses on evening [shift], and three nurses on night shift. There was no way that I could take care of all this. So I said, "Okay, well, let's do data, data, data, and that's what everybody wants." So we pulled the data. For example, we used to give about one magnesium [supplement] run a month. We were giving seven a day, so we went from once a month to 35 a month.

B: These were the kind of statistics that you were putting in there?

P: Yes, so I said, "Okay, we will build our case. We need to let them know that where nursing time [was] maybe 15 minutes out of the hour [before the more acute patients arrived,] it's now 45 minutes out of the hour in that room. Obviously, if you are in that room, you can't be inside other rooms. We put our proposal together, and it was overwhelmingly received; it was, "Yes, you can have what you need." That was a really good win. They realized that it wasn't that the staff didn't want to work hard; this [new patient acuity] was beyond what they could do.

B: Yes, you couldn't succeed at what you were doing unless you had that addition; you provided the documentation, so they could back you up.

P: And leadership was really supportive. That was probably the single most important thing. Until this day they continue to recognize, and we continue to look at, those numbers because the patients aren't getting any better. They are incredible, acute, complex patients.

B: Absolutely. They need that staffing to be able to give them the care that they need.

P: Right. That was probably one of the real important pieces that I've seen from the leadership.

B: In speaking of leadership, you haven't mentioned mentors. Have you had a mentor in this setting?

P: That probably is the only thing that has not been the greatest experience. And that's because I've had five bosses in ten years. So roughly every two years my boss leaves or is promoted or something.

B: You are talking about clinical directors?

P: Yes, T. was here about nine years and now it's R. T. has been here the entire time that I have been a manager up until January; then R. took over in January. The VP has been solid, but it's the clinical directors that have changed. One became a VP in another system hospital. The other one, I don't know what she did; I think she went to do consulting work. The other one [left] because they revamped [our organizational structure]; our hospital is constantly growing, so they changed how they were going to break sections down into surgical sections, critical care sections, and things like that. I haven't had a really strong mentor here.

B: At any other point in your career?

P: No, the last mentor I had was someone whom I did not like. I knew how I didn't want to be the boss by the way that person was the boss.

B: So that person wasn't a mentor—more like a corrective example.

P: Yes.

B: Have you had anybody who showed you the ropes or who was a champion for you?

P: Not really. I think just having the forums that we have here with regard to our unit director meetings. Because I am a multilevel unit director, I also sit on the nurse executive group, so [that means] just being exposed to the same people. Although not always my boss all of the time, I kind of collectively had pieces of mentoring, I guess. I've kind of taken pieces of how people do things, what I like, and I try to emulate that. There have been examples.

B: I call it exemplars rather than mentors. So nobody took your side or was watching or you felt was watching out for you or [served as] a really ongoing role model. Rather, you looked around at different people—what they did, either positive or negative—and said, "I'm going to do something like that." You have been learning from your experience and building a kind of leadership model from what you have seen around you, it seems.

P: I have. Most of these questions all seem very positive and proactive. . . . But I see that other unit directors whom I work with are feeling and being over-whelmed because they don't have good mentorship, either. I do think there needs to be someone, needs to be mentoring, because not everybody can sur-vive [without it]. I am not patting myself on the back. I just think it's because I am a little bit older than most of the other unit directors. I had ten years of management before I came into nursing; I think that has helped me. I have vari-ous things in my personal life that really ground me that [are lacking for] some of the newer unit directors [who] are struggling, and I see that.

B: You can look at that and see. That is a strength that you have to learn from your experience, whether because of your religious upbringing or what happened in your family or previous management job, or because of just looking around at some of your colleagues here. Tell me about this organization. This particular organization—how has this been a good fit in enhancing your success?

P: There are years and years of experience in these walls. People stay here forever. . . . Yes, there are some people who stay because this is all they know, but there are also people who stay here because they like it, and there are also people who stay here because they feel they make a difference. I tend to believe that a lot of people stay here because of that. I have nurses who work for me who have been here for 30 years on this same unit. Their knowledge is invalu-able; they've seen a lot come and go—and that is really neat. I probably have one of the older, tenured staff in the building. I think nurses [here] are hardy. I think they are more outspoken and they will speak their minds. And they are incred-ibly gifted, confident, and skilled staff that you don't see everywhere—that com-bination of those skills. We do a lot of things like going for Magnet status, but even before we did that, we always felt that we had that stature. We had a great reputation for nursing even before we started talking about Magnet [status]. It [comes from] years of being very focused and centered in the community.

I think, just building on that, the history of nursing at [institution name omit-ted] has always been very valued, and even [what] we learned in nursing school, which is really nice. It shows new people coming into the organization that we are committed to our organization and we are committed to the ongoing foster-ing, networking, and growing of good nurses.

B: Yes, [you have] a long-standing reputation of commitment and of education. All those things are a good fit for you. The next question has to do with a time when you were supported by your organization. You talked earlier how the organization helped you succeed by adding the staff that you needed to meet the patient's needs. Did you have another particular example of support from your organization?

P: I think we have a lot of little things that continue to show the support of the organization. We do a lot of different things. We have a tea cart that comes to the staff for tea breaks, for staff who can't go off the unit. It has chocolates and apples and hot tea. We do something called quiet time every day at 2:00, where we shut down the lights in the hallways and dim the lights in the nurses station for that half-hour from 2:00 to 2:30, so that nurses can regroup in their day. You are supposed to try to be quiet and only talk when you need to talk.

B: Is it enforced?

P: It pretty much is. If you go in units, you will see the lights all dimmed low. During Christmastime, people brought Christmas CDs and then they brought their own favorite music instead of something very relaxing. I let them listen to whatever they want to listen to, because it's their quiet time. If that's what they want to listen to, then that is fine with me. We have senior nurses recognition days, for nurses who have over five years of [service as] a nurse. Of course, Nurses Week is always a big deal around here. The VP of nursing and nurse executive group come in and do night rounds a couple of times a year to meet with the night staff.

So there are a lot of little things that we do. It's probably something monthly that recognizes that you are doing a good job or we're looking at your role as a nurse. Whether it's letting us give them 12-hour shifts, or letting us do a weekend program, we are always looking at what we can do to recruit and retain our most valued resource, our nurses.

B: To make your lives better, to help you rejuvenate, to recognize you—all those things, you experience that as support. Now the fantasy question: Let's say that behind you is a whole room of new nurse managers, and you get to wish three things for them to ensure that they will be in their job at least as long as you have and they will be as successful in it as you have been. What would you wish for them to help make that happen?

P: I would wish strong mentorship for them. I think that would be very important. I would also wish for them that there would be an equitable balance in job expectations. What I mean by that is some managers manage an 8-bed unit and others manage a 57-bed unit. The expectations are the same, and that is not fair; there is not a good balance. I know that different units have different needs, and it's not always about numbers, but I think there needs to be some kind of balance. Maybe the manager who manages the 8-bed unit has to sit on three committees so that the one who manages the [57-bed unit] doesn't. There has to be a better balance, because if we don't do something, then you're going to have the manager say, "Well, I'm going to do three twelves [3 days of 12-hour shifts] then, and let someone else do this."

B: Because they have a 3-day, 12-hour shift in another hospital.

P: Or even at this hospital. You need to be able to recruit and retain good managers as well. You have to do some of the things that you see in other industries, like maybe four tens [4 days of 10-hour shifts]. Or every other Friday you have an office day or you can leave by noon or something. I kid my staff that the one who has the worst schedule on the whole unit is me. Everybody else has got it pretty nice. There has to be a piece that managers need to be able to feel like they should be able to put their request out there on the table as well. Those are my three wishes, I guess.

B: I got two. When did you go to three, because one was the mentorship and second was the equity of taking the look at what you are really doing?

P: The third would be more go out into industry and use some of the successful tools they've used for their managers, whether it's a dress-down Friday in some places or get some flexible scheduling. Or, we all have computer access at home, so why could we not work one day or two days a month at home?

B: So you picked the pockets of some industry-standard companies that have been successful at their managerial level and do the same here. And the techniques that you're looking to borrow—are they a certain kind or do they add more work–life balance? Because the example you gave was that. We are picking their pockets, and what are you looking for?

P: I think I am looking for a couple of things. I'm looking for work–life balance. This really doesn't pertain to me, because I really get fulfillment from what I do. I get it from my staff. I get it from the "thank you" note board—I get it from that. There are people who feel that they need to be told if they do a good job, but not only told that, but shown that in some way, like a parker [parking-oriented reward] of some sort.

B: Like a parking spot? So [your third wish is that] we get some other ideas from business and industry on rewarding people and making them feel important, making their lives easier, giving them better work–life balance. We borrow some of those ideas and apply them.

P: We did start a program of [incentivizing] the middle manager [who met] certain goals in a fiscal year. We would get so much of a dollar amount for meeting our goals. [That program] has been very successful. We started that last year. I don't know of too many other nurse groups that are doing that.

B: That is interesting. No, this is the first time I've heard that, so that is one of those definite examples. It's applied from another arena to this arena.

P: I'm curious to see, since I manage two units, if my goals will be based on both ends or not.

B: Maybe you can combine them. The last question: You are driving home tonight and you slip through a wrinkle in time. It is ten years from now, and we are not hearing about nurse managers leaving their jobs. They are satisfied. They are staying for ten years or more. What would have to happen between now and 2016 for this to be the case?

P: I would say that those managers are working for leadership that has provided a work–home balance. Because that's what everybody is saying today, that is what everybody wants. They want to be able to have time with their families. Ever since September 11 [the terrorist attacks in 2001], you see that more and more people have just regrouped.

The other piece of that is, as you get older and you get life experiences, things start to change. What you thought was important isn't important. You start to get a little more philosophical in your life—I think that is just normal. What was important when I was 20 is not as important when I'm 40. I think in this year 2015 we would say that we somehow have been able to balance a nurse manager's workload more effectively and have done some of those things that keep a person in place ten years, because that is not the case anymore. When I recruit, I recruit a nurse for two years. I don't even go down that path because everybody comes in with [certain expectations]. These nurses today, when they're 20 years old, they know what they want: I am going to do this for one year, and do this, and get my master's, et cetera. They have it all at 20 years old; they have it all figured out. It took me until 31 to decide if I even wanted to go into nursing. It's amazing that you are not going to have—I would never have—a staff member for 30 years again, never. It's not how the thinking is today. It's this: "I want it now and if I don't get it here, then I'm going here." It's not an automaton thing.

B: Given that, that is the generation coming. What would it take for this generation to be there for ten years? Let's say someone in that generation gets that job tomorrow.

P: Well, why would you go work with the unit and take care of six, seven, or ten patients at night when you can go work in ICU and take care of two?

B: I don't know. What's the answer?

P: I don't know the answer. That's our problem today. Years ago, you didn't allow nurses to take care of somebody in the ICU until they had five years of experience on a medical/surgical floor. Now they're recruited right out of nursing school. [In the past,] you couldn't get a specialty to save your soul. I think the answer is that the bedside nurse should be paid the most, not the ICU nurse.

The bedside nurse handles the most geography, handles the most patients, and doesn't have half the resources that an ICU nurse has. So I think you need to put the money on the bedside and not in the ICU.

B: What about the money for the nurse manager?

P: Well, that always should be higher, I think. I mean, . . . there are people in my staff taking home more money in a week than I am, based on the hours. There are some nurses not too far below me on an hourly rate.

B: So if we circle back to this ideal that it's 2015 and nurse managers are staying, how does money figure into that?

P: I think it's figured in at some point—it has to. A lot of money has been poured into nursing now, [in the form of] recruitments, forgiveness loans, and tuition reimbursement. There are a lot of programs to recruit and retain nurses. You would need to do the same kind of longevity plan or some type of retention for nurse management. And not even for just nurse managers, but to keep a nurse on a unit for 5, 10, or 15 years as well. Business does it. I hate to think it's all about money, and I don't think it's all about money, but the reality is that there is a factor in the money.

B: Is there anything else you want to add to that question?

P: I think that we have to constantly look at the acuity of the patient. We have to assure, not only for the nurse, but also for the patient, that we continue to make good choices on how we staff units and be real diligent in monitoring that. I don't know if I'm fortunate or unfortunate. If my staff calls me at 8:00 at night and says, "It's really pretty bad here, and our numbers say we should downsize a nurse," and I'll say, "If you are telling me it's pretty bad, then you keep that nurse. You are the one who is there assessing the situation; I am at home. If you really believe you need to keep that nurse, then you keep that nurse and we will deal with the outcome later." I think we trust nurses with people's lives, but we don't always trust some of the decisions that they make. I think that has to go away to a degree. If someone is calling me and telling me, "It's really bad here right now; we need to keep that body here," then you do it and I tell them to do it. I have been really fortunate every time we've done it. It has not come back to hit us, and that tells me that they are making good decisions. They are making the right decisions—and sometimes the right decision isn't the popular decision. That's what has to happen sometimes.

B: In the context of this question, that would mean one way to keep nurse managers in place is for people to recognize your authority, while you, in turn, down the line, recognize the authority of a staff nurse.

P: Right. Because then you are cultivating future managers. If you are starting to help them to make decisions, then that's only beneficial to the group at large.

B: Right—that's the whole culture model you said like: "Okay, you have a problem. What are you going to do about it?" You were talking about cultivating managers, yet you would say, "I hired these nurses and I'm looking at them, thinking they will probably be here for two years." How do you do both?

P: Well, that's the hard part. I don't know. What I try to do is, I say, "touch them." I still try to always keep my pulse on what they think and what they want—but you don't. I have to realize that it's not me; it's them. I can't take it seriously. I can put the same amount of energy and focus and time and work into two different people, and one may stay five years and one may go in a year. [Their decision does not reflect] what I have given. I have to know that at the end of the day, when I look in the mirror, I did the best I could with what I had and that's what I do and that is how I work. Not every manager is comfortable with that. They feel like a failure. I don't feel that way. I am telling the VP of nursing every chance I get that these people are not staying anymore. We need to figure out something different. It's not enough to say, "Oh, let's give them the weekend program." Some want that, but not everybody wants that.

B: At the end of the day, it sounds like you are doing the best that you can, but there are factors outside [at play; you are] not taking it personally, so it worked.

P: You have to. If I didn't, I wouldn't be here for my nurses. You are tough skinned, because you get it from the top and you get it from the staff. To end this, I always say I have the nicest group of selfish people you ever wanted to work for. Because "It's all about me"—that is all you hear them say. It's all about them. It's what they want, when they want it, and how they want it. They are nice about it, but that is what it's about.

B: Meeting their needs, you mean?

P: Yes, they'll say, "I know that we have to work a holiday, but I really want to be off for Christmas." All 55 of them want to be off Christmas. I'll say, "Okay, we'll just shut the unit for Christmas. What do you think?" It's not going to happen. Or they'll say, "I want to work this schedule," "I want to work that schedule," et cetera. I tell them, "Take your schedule and fill it in. Just make sure you are covered—you can do whatever you want." They say, "Oh, no, you do it." It's amazing, but yet they are the nicest group of people. They expect me to kind of balance all that. That's the hard part. I am kind of tired of that piece of it.

B: What was it like for you, answering these questions?

P: I wrote notes and things, but I didn't spend a whole lot of time with that.

B: Yes, what was the interview process for you in terms of answering the questions?

P: I thought it was easier because I thought this would be a teleconference. I didn't think it was going to be one-on-one like this. I like this better because I'm not the most gifted when it comes to putting words together. You were able to reiterate back to me what I was saying, which validated if that was what I was saying, so I like that interaction. I could say, "Yes, I agree" or "No, that's not what I meant to say." That part being one-on-one was really comfortable. I like that better.

B: Good. It was interesting that you expected something different. It's a distance, but did you discover or observe anything about yourself while we were talking? How did you seem to yourself as you talked about and reflected on your work?

P: When I talk about what I do and the people I work with, it stirs that passion that I have in nursing and [emphasizes] how important it is to me. Because when you lose the passion, it's time to get the heck out of it. I always feel rejuvenated at the time when the most difficult questions have to be asked or when a challenge to come up with an answer or solution to a problem [is posed.] That is why I choose to do what I'm doing.

B: That's so wonderful to end on. For my part, what I want to say is that my observation is that you have this passion of "It's all about the patients." You have this enormous respect for the expertise of people whom you work with and their own power that informs your power and your decision making. You are a really keen observer of yourself, and you can learn lessons from looking around you—everything from what you learned in a more of a business kind of managerial setting to looking around at the different leaders and saying "Yes" or "No." You have a really good ability to take your life experience and make that wisdom borne of experience, some positive and some not so positive, but just take that and learn from it. But it's always about the patient for you. Your most animated times are talking about them—"It's about the patients" times—but also when you are talking about your real gratitude and recognition of how great your staff is and what they do.

P: They are.

B: Yes, even when they are asking for [time off for] Christmas, Thanksgiving, Memorial Day, or whatever else it is. It has been great to talk to you, and I thank you for being so open about your experiences. Of course, we are looking for trends, but each person is a unique gem, so it was great to just talk to you.

P: Thank you. I was very honored to be selected. That was nice.

Transcript of Full Interview

All identifiers have been removed to protect confidentiality. This exuberant manager sought a management role because of her interest in how things work. She expresses her ardor in her frequent and unexpected use of the word "fun." Note that her positive framework driven by seeking—and finding—her staff's best intentions. In this way, she creates an optimism that is equal parts resilient thinking and self-restraint. She mirrors the generativity and mission focus of her organization.

Use this interview transcript for your own research as a case study or as a discussion focus in class. As you read, try to identify the signature strengths of the individual nurse manager being interviewed as well as the strengths of her organization.

B = Interviewer

P = Participant

B: Let's start with your beginnings as a middle manager. When you think about your first impressions that were satisfying and promising in the first few weeks, we'll probably have to go back to when you were in the acting manager role.

P: It was different, you know. There was a definite difference between being acting manager and being the manager.

B: I think you're right about that. If you can, tell me about when you had the designated job.

P: When I actually got the job for real.

B: What were the things that held promise or were positive and satisfying in the first few months of having the role?

P: I have been a staff nurse on this unit, and then I've been an assistant nurse manager, and then I've been an acting nurse manager. I loved getting out to the other areas in the hospital and seeing how other things worked. I notice that other people sometimes figure that stuff out on their own, but I never did. To me, things are a black hole until I've gotten down there and have seen how things work. I guess I didn't ever really wonder about it, either. I mean some things, I had no idea what happened—like prior to surgery once they left here. Things like that. It was just very fun for me to see the way the rest of the hospital worked.

I can just remember, I was a staff nurse and we had a materials management guy who had his father here. I just had no idea what his job was—you know what I mean? Unless you deliver stuff, I can't even fathom what you do. I just loved that. I thought that was really fun, and that's part of the reason that I was interested in the role—just for the backdrop of it.

I took the job when our unit was at 50% staffing. It was in a major crisis. My director said, "I couldn't in good conscience give this job to you, because you're a brand-new manager and this is a horrible situation," and I talked her into hiring me anyway. Well, you know, you can go one way or another, and I decided to go for it. [The director] actually had interviewed a really, really experienced manager, but who said she would only be here for two years. That's fine, but I told her, "You don't want to go with somebody who has more experience but will be gone in two years. I'll be here in two years and I'll have experience by then." I really did want it. I was very positive about it in general. I knew the unit and I knew the problems.

The other things that made it so positive to me were I liked being out there, I liked working with the staff, and I liked the idea of getting their ideas and trying to put them into place. I'm not the kind of person who cares about me coming up with the idea or me getting the credit for anything. I just really like to have [my staff] feel that satisfaction that something they thought of got done. Occasionally I'll have a big opinion or idea that I'll try to push through with it. It's not really my modus operandi.

It was a hard time, but it was also fun. It's nice to look back and say, "We did that."

B: A couple of things that I want to go back on: You were attracted to what some people would have thought as a really tough situation.

P: I thought it would come around. I saw it would come around because I had been on this unit when it was well functioning before the nursing shortage started. And I just figured it would get back to that—and it has.

B: On one hand, you had some kind of institutional memory of being able to do that. But what about you: Do you see that as making you think you could do it?

P: There is something about the actual job. I loved being a floor nurse, but there's something about the way my brain works that I would always try to think of the ways that you can organizationally make things better for people. I felt like was getting to do more of the stuff that I enjoyed. This is the funny part. I even enjoyed doing—and back then I really did not do a bunch of it—personnel disciplinary stuff. Because I really—and this is not too different to me than taking care of patients—I really like to take an icky situation and try to help the person see it. I treat them with respect and dignity, and let them leave feeling like they feel okay about it, even if I just told them, "Well, you can't work here anymore." I still want them to feel like they were treated well and that they can see that maybe it was better for them or whatever. That doesn't always work out, obviously. But I think it's a fun challenge. It felt like I was really learning more when I did stuff like that and I like to learn a lot.

There's something about the nurses having to juggle so many things. I liked it when I got to be an RN3 and then acting nurse manager. I liked the feeling that you had this stuff to work on, and it would still be here tomorrow. It sounds gross really, when you think about it in another way, but I would feel terrible if I forgot to bring somebody back a straw that they asked me for. I had a lot of feelings like that. I was forgetting stuff on the floor—you know what I mean? With this type of job, I feel a little more successful. Does that make sense?

B: Yes. What's the difference, though, because surely at the end of every day you can go, "Okay, what did I forget today?"

P: It doesn't feel that way to me anymore. Maybe it's my attitude, I don't know. Not to say I didn't, say, feel successful on the floor, because I did and I loved it, I really did. I thought I was pretty good with patients and stuff. Then I got to be the assistant nurse manager. When I went from being RN3 to being an acting director, I just really felt that there is hard stuff to do, because as an RN3, I have three RN3s, and I give them all kinds of props. You have to go from being a charge nurse one day to being in the office another, and then go back to being charge and trying to remember what you were trying to carry forward. I am just not good at that. You can feel when you are not pulling your strings. I did it, but I always was wondering, "What am I supposed to be remembering?" I don't feel like that in this job. I guess I could have a day here or there where I forgot something, but for the most part I feel like it's a little bit more planned over time. I can decide some things can be done today and some things can be done next week. I can take a little more time to think about it. It just fits my personality better.

B: We're going to talk about that in a minute. I just want to follow up with one question, and then I want to talk about that sense that this role is a better fit and it played to your strengths. Can you talk about anything that you learned during that early time that helped you succeed? And I'm going to say one thing—that you just told me that this job is a better fit for you and you are feeling less this sense of something got left behind and that's not a good feeling. You're sort of more haunted by the feeling that somehow you were not doing a good job. But one of the things that you learned in that early time is, "This fits; I can get the sense of a job well done and not a lot of stragglers left behind." Is there anything else you learned? What were you going to say?

P: Well, it's hard to feel like you have a job well done. But it's not the same kind of little nagging feeling. You know what I mean? It felt like I had still left things undone, but it wasn't the same as it used to be. And actually I'm pretty okay with it; I don't know how to describe it. If you look on a personality test, it would say the same thing. I'm okay with things being open, wide open, and things don't have to be. I'm not a list person particularly, although I have to write things down. I'm okay with vagueness or ambiguity. To me, the job was like, "There are all these things I could be working on." You just pick and work on things at different times, and things have their time. Maybe people are upset about something but nobody else is, but then two or three different areas get upset about it. Then it's "Okay, time to take that one on." I feel pretty comfortable with "loosey goosey." Maybe what was super-important yesterday is totally not important today. It doesn't bother me. I see that as different from my peers.

B: Okay, we'll talk about that in a little bit. Your peers in this role?

P: Or just in nursing—it's like, "Doesn't that just drive you crazy?" [For me,] not really. There are things that drive other people crazy; they just don't drive me crazy.

B: And one of them is a tolerance for uncertainty or ambiguity or lack of clarity?

P: Or the fact that things take a while to happen. I have less control than people would want, I think, sometimes.

B: Of being willing to just say, "I have limited control; I have influence but not control."

P: What I really feel like is, it'll come around eventually, if it's really important. I have limited control but I get to review a lot.

B: You also have some kind of almost optimism, even starting from "Well, this unit is really down but I can remember when it wasn't."

P: I'm incredibly optimistic. I am always optimistic. I always am.

B: Just even starting with the way you took on this role—the way things were, but you were thinking it would come around.

P: Now what were you asking me right before that? I kind of went off on a tangent.

B: No, actually you were answering the question: What you learned during that time. Mostly what you're saying is that you learned a lot about yourself.

P: The other thing I would answer to that question is that I learned how important it is to have a network within the hospital, just to get to know as many people as possible. That always pays off in the long run. And [it's important] to help people when you can, because you're going to ask them for help later. To not think, "Well, I don't like that person." You just say, "I'm going to like everybody; I'm going to work with everybody." To me, that's incredibly important. One of the nicest things that my director did for me was say, "You need to go out and meet with everybody in every department." Any department that we interface with, I went and talked to its director. It was people whom I actually don't interface with in my role that much. They were probably only a step above, but I didn't know that. I was talking to the director of Patient Data Services. I never talk to [that person]. But at least at one time I met [the director]—that person has retired since then. I found out what [the director's] point of view was about what was needed from me and what the goals were for that department. I went all over the place.

B: One of the things you learned in that early period—and it was spurred on by your director—was the importance of interconnecting and reciprocity, even if it wasn't someone who was in your view at the time.

P: I also think it's important to know that we're doing this and they're doing this, and they're related—but they're different and their goals are different. [Then] we all have to have in mind what they're trying to do and how that can be played for both people's advantage at different times.

B: And their piece of it. You were talking about how cool it was to sort of get there and find out what people were doing out there. You got a real excitement about the big picture. Let's talk about your view of the positive factors influencing you to stay in your job. Everyone who is part of the study has been at the job for at least five years—and that's not as easy to find as you might think. So the question for you is, "What are the positive factors in you and in this organization that have allowed you to stay in the role?"

P: The key thing—well, I don't know if this is the key thing, but one really major thing if it hadn't happened I probably wouldn't be here—is that we have kind of pulled out of that staffing doldrums that we were in when I started the role. We went from having 19.5 FTEs [full-time equivalent employees], we probably budgeted for about 30 at that time or something. We are now budgeted for 40 to 45 or something and we have 43 [FTEs]. So we've gone from having 19 to 43 RN FTEs at the present time. If I hadn't been able to do that, I wouldn't feel successful.

B: Straightforward "being able to get the staffing that you needed."

P: So many things come along with that—I mean, you can just imagine. So many things come along with that. Put a huge focus on the orientation programs so you can bring that many nurses in. Some years we were bringing 18 nurses in one year. This is an incredibly high-acuity unit. And to orient that many people for 12 weeks. It was a huge task on the unit, but it almost became like the norm; it became part of our daily work. Anyway, that was part of it.

When we nose-dived staffing-wise, we lost all of our professional practice staff. We had nurse practice committees and scheduling committees, and the people would quit, and you couldn't get someone else to join it. We didn't have the staffing to support somebody leaving the unit for a meeting. As our staffing has gotten better, as hard as that was, those things come back to life. Then you say, "This is a fun job." You start your quality committee again; your people are doing projects; you know you can support nurses in doing presentations and posters. It's like a whole other layer. We knew back then that we were in survival mode. You know it when you're in it, but you've got to build back out of it. If that hadn't happened . . . I mean, it's not just staffing, it's just the whole culture.

B: What other factors do you think there are?

P: There are so many factors. Another factor is that I love working with these nurses. I just have a really smart group of nurses to work with. We have a great staff. I have three RN3s, which makes this job a total pleasure. . . . They each have their own stuff they do. I am here to support them. I am not bogged down in so much of the day-to-day [details, but] I can see that some of my peers are. For example, one of my RN3s has one day a week of management, and occasionally I will give her more if she needs it. She organizes the orientation program, and she does the schedule with some help. She also does a preceptor workshop every year and works with the preceptors and does the orientation schedules and talks to the preceptors—she does the whole thing. And one of them [the RN3s] does all the work with all the nursing assistants and the monitor technicians and the patient–family education and their meeting. They [all of the RN3s] have stuff they do.

B: They have stuff that they do that you might be doing?

P: But you know what? It plays to their strengths. They do it. I am ultimately accountable for it, but I'm just here to help them if they need help.

B: Back to you for factors: For you, part of [the reason for your success] is just [the nurses'] excellence, but also they get themselves involved in a sense of a team?

P: And I think the structure works.

B: Structure?

P: The way we have work divided out.

B: So nobody is as overwhelmed and burdened with so many different things.

P: The other thing that happened was that in 2000, our CNO brought in a new position, an operations supervisor. She does payroll and administrative duties that I used to do. I used to do that all the time; I used to be in total paperwork hell all the time.

B: A general theme here is that in some ways, the roles are divided. Though you might have oversight, there are a lot of things that someone else is doing so that in your role, you're wearing a lot of hats but not as many as you were.

P: Right, and we have a lot of clarity, [in case] somebody [has a question] about who's doing what and what the roles are. If somebody comes up with a question about CPR, I know exactly who she's going to talk to. Some things are me, and some things are them.

B: Let's just talk about you. This has become the classically uncomfortable question. We've touched on some of this, which is great. What gifts, values, attitudes, and capabilities do you bring to the challenge of the nurse management role, and how have these qualities allowed you to be successful and work long term in this role? We have touched on optimism, attraction to challenge, seeing the big picture.

P: I like that. I think the biggest thing that I think about—and I don't know if anybody would even know that I think about this, but I do think about it—is when I try to maintain and be optimistic and nonjudgmental.

B: Let's take that apart. What does it feel like?

P: I'm not going to get bogged down or discouraged very easily. We'll have five new nurses and somebody's fighting with someone else and then something's not going well and some of my group will be disgusted and frustrated and "This is never going to work" and "Oh my God!" You can think of so many examples where people think, "This is never going to work; this unit is going down the tank." When people get like that, I feel like one of the things that I offer is to say, "It's not that bad, you know. Let's just try to objectify it. Let's try to depersonalize it and pick up and go from here. What do we really want to happen? What will really help us get there? You know, all these feelings aren't really going to help. If you can let some of that go, [we can] move forward and set some new goals. Maybe they'll be smaller, or [maybe we'll have] a little struggle with something." I feel like I do that all the time. And I do it with my peers, also: "It's alright. You know what? Things like this happen, and it's not that out of the ordinary. Let's just take a deep breath and think about what we want to have happen." I try not to dwell on the past.

A nurse came up to me and said, "Oh, this family—there's 40 people in this person's family and they are totally blocking us. If we have to do CPR, we'd be in a predicament." My response was, "How wonderful this person has 40 people here to see them. You need to open your mind. My family is a big family, and we [also] do that." That's my background, anyway: My whole family just invades. "The patient has support, [so we need to focus on what] we need to do to help them."

That's just one example of trying not to judge: "Just don't go there. We're not here for that, you know . . . we're here to provide nursing care." Nursing care is not about judging the patient, the family, your peers—it's not about that.

B: You introduced this by saying, "I don't know if people would know this, but I think about it all the time." Your idea of being nonjudgmental has components of optimism with expectations that it will work out. It has elements of collaboration, but also I want to capture this other essence. It's a little bit of "big picture" thinking and it's always "operate with the end in mind."

P: That is so true. I treat people like they had the best of intentions, [even] if they didn't. Actually, I just think that way; that's just how I think. But I do it intentionally, too. If somebody does something that seems counterproductive to the team, I see it as "You were trying to help that patient, weren't you?" I'll give them a way to [explain their actions so that] they can show that they had good intentions, whether or not it was true. Sometimes I get them to think that it was true.

B: You give them a way to understand that "the best may have been lurking."

P: That's exactly right. That opens them up, so they are going to talk to me. My end result is I want them to improve; that's my end result. When I first started, I had an RN3, and it was just her and me. We couldn't be more opposite. She was wonderful in her way, but she couldn't do that. . . . She would just be so down on somebody. I said, "You want to yell at them because they did something wrong, but it is not going to get what you want from that person. It might feel right and you can say, 'I'm totally justified in being mad,' but what does that get you? You want the person to feel like you're on their side and you want them to go from here to here. There's nothing to gain from yelling at someone and, not literally yelling at someone, but just scolding them." And there is a tendency to go to that.

I think it's real important to remember what is it that you're trying to do. What are you trying to accomplish? If you're trying to help [nurses] grow, scolding them is never going to make it. That goes back to me being a nurse in a really awful patient care situation. . . . Our acting manager was helping out because somebody had left, and she treated me like I hadn't done anything wrong. She treated me the positive way. She treated me like, "Well, what could you do here?" I had a patient who should have been in the ICU; I was really new and I was floundering, and she [the acting manager] didn't treat me like an idiot. She treated me like, "This is what you had—tell me what you had? Of course, that makes perfect sense. You could have used this; you could have used that." I really could have. It wasn't a super-great moment of my practice. I was getting support and help, but she treated me like she was talking to herself or a good friend. That's how I try to treat people.

B: [The acting manager] and that behavior became a kind of model for you, and one of the components of [that model is that] you assume that the person is trying to do their best. You don't judge them.

P: And you assume that they want to continue to improve. I always try—and I think I am pretty good at it—I try to figure out what could have been motivating them at that time or what they might have been thinking. I try to get to know everybody, but especially my own staff, as well as I can and know what kind of things that make them excited. I try really hard to just think where they might be coming from.

B: So it's that reversibility—like stepping into their shoes. All these are elements of being nonjudgmental. I've never quite heard it said that way, but it's really true as you talk about it. There are all these different elements that actually go into the moment where you are being nonjudgmental. That's a really great anatomy of it, and that along with the other parts are some really key strengths. Can you think of anything else, of things that you bring to the role?

P: I think that's my underlying thing. I wish I could work more. I'm very, very liberal and I don't talk about that at work either. But how are you going to [put in] your two cents to help the world? I try to hire people with different backgrounds, and that's gotten me in trouble. But you just keep on trying to [put in] your two cents the best way you can, you know? We don't have enough nurses of different backgrounds, so I'm going to try to find them and bring them in. I'm going to try to be nondiscriminatory. I'm going to try to help people to be more understanding of each other. I really want to bring in more cultural stuff to the unit. It makes me feel like I'm doing something that relates to my values.

B: What you're saying is that you are trying to be congruent with the values that you have outside this place and bring them back to work in a way that feels comfortable enough to do that.

P: It helps, I think. Having that attitude helps people who are discongruent [understand] that they could see positives in each other. I feel like I've helped with that over the years.

B: That brings me to the next question, which in a way you've been in the process of answering in so many ways. I just want to put it out there as a whole question. It's the people aspect. It's such a big cast of characters with whom you have to communicate—patients, patients' families, nurses, organizational people, administrators, directors. What particular thing do you bring to the role that allows you to connect with so many different kinds of people? We talked about elements of being nonjudgmental, being able to try and put yourself in their position. Is there something that you wanted to underline or something else here that we haven't covered that you want to add?

P: I think those are the big parts. One more piece of it is that I love working here and I love taking care of patients, and that's important, too. If you are going to talk to somebody, I think it always helps if we can bond on that. We're here to take care of the patients, and we're going to do whatever we need to do for them. I think that kind of rounds it out. Does that make sense?

B: The idea that you have a common purpose, regardless of the personality differences or the variation in roles. Your working assumption is "We're all here for the same reason."

P: Right. If you treat people like that, even if they weren't in that place at that moment, it helps you bring the conversation to a higher level. It may sound a little manipulative.

B: No, not at all. It reminds me of your other really core positives of treating people as looking for their best intentions. Isn't it an example of that? Let's talk about that. You say, "I want to go into this and communicate the sense that we are all doing this for the patient," and you treat people that way. Can you think of an incident where you did that?

P: Basically it would be, if I was going to work with somebody who doesn't know much about our unit. I could think of working with somebody in Materials

Management or something. I would start with a story that shows them what it means to the patient here so that the context would be set.

B: You mean what their work means to the patient?

P: Right. Whatever the conflict is, whatever the problem is, I would make sure that it was just framed in such a way that they could see how important it is.

B: I'm just trying to figure out how that works. Have you done that? I'm just trying to think [of how] somebody comes in here from one department and you explain how we're all in this together because you're doing this really important thing.

P: Well, I always like to have a context, especially if somebody is asking for something or making a change. Basically, all I'm doing is setting the context. If I'm saying, "We really need these urinals here," that's too obvious, because everybody knows that. It would be more like starting from the beginning—just saying, "We've got these patients. I need this thing, and nurses try to get it. When they can't get it, they get frustrated and it takes time away from other patients. I know that's what you're trying to do, too—trying to get things for patients. So what do we need to do to improve this process?"

B: That's another aspect of it—communicating context and shared purpose somehow, and actually putting that into words and not just thinking it.

P: You can be funny, you know. You can just imagine somebody sitting in the middle of the hallway waiting [to use a urinal]. It just gives you a lot of chances to lighten the atmosphere, and it makes it real obvious what needs to happen sometimes.

B: And takes away any of that kind of defensiveness.

P: That is exactly what I'm thinking of, too. You don't want to be accused of [that.] I like to be honest and at the same time have them not feel stung by it. Because we have our problems, too; it's not like everything works perfectly on this unit.

B: "Here's what we need and why, and if we all do this, we can get to X."

P: And "You guys have been doing such a great job of focusing on this, I wonder if you forgot about this."

B: Again, that's your positive framing. Let's go to what's satisfying and gratifying about this role and your contribution that gives you a feeling of pride. With all these questions, the longer we talk, the more you will have touched on some of them. But for you, what makes this [the nurse manager role] satisfying?

P: It is just a really juicy setting, because we've got really sick patients and, for the nurses, we try to hire the smartest people we can. Our nurses are just so bright. They go from being a new graduate to running a committee by themselves or going to great lengths to make something different for a patient and figuring stuff out. We get to recognize people and present them awards toward things. To see that growth is one of the best parts of the job.

To have visible improvements in how the workload goes—it's still heavy, I mean it's just heavy. Ten months ago or . . . maybe a year ago, . . . we improved our staffing by a whole number, so the nurses on day shift only take three patients. We went from having four [patients per nurse] to taking three. It's a huge improvement, [and I] feel like things are getting better all the time. I can look at the nurse and say, "I'm here to support you; that's my role." And to have them be able to see things get better, to say they enjoy the educational things, [is very gratifying.]

Now here's the one thing I give up: I don't get credit for many things, which is okay with me. If something exciting happens, probably one of my RN3s or one of the RN2s is going to get the credit. I just sit back and enjoy that. I think it's wonderful. I just love to see that growth.

B: So it's accomplishing through people doing a job.

P: Yes, and having them feel like things are positive. We're proud of this unit. People want to come here. People floating around say, "Wow, you guys really have your act together. Nobody else ever asked me if I had lunch yet, but you guys always do." Stuff like that.

B: It's not so much taking the credit, but rather the gratification of having created that kind of environment with those kinds of things along with everybody else here.

P: We've all created it. But yes, that's it.

B: It's a really different kind of contribution than if you had every one of the staff nurses who was part of all this. You create the atmosphere and frame it.

P: To think as creatively as possible, to try to get that.

B: You didn't mention creativity as one of the things that you value about yourself. Talk about that. We'll just backtrack for a moment.

P: I try not to think [follow] the standard line. I go out here and look at things.

B: In general, what's your thought process? Each situation is different. If it's not, if your inner little dialogue isn't "what we've always done," then what is?

P: I think, "We could do this or we could do that"—just trying to think of something or brainstorming. Both of my parents are in nursing leadership, and my mother will tell me things I could do and she will throw out some totally crazy ideas. Maybe we wouldn't even want that, but it opens up the minds of everybody, I think.

B: There's a name for that which I love—it's "constraint-free analysis." It's sort of like "Here's the problem, but what if . . . ?" Some of this stuff is way out there. There's a real sense in you that there was a lot of modeling in your family of some of the things that you see here.

P: That's probably why when I was an RN2, I was thinking about that stuff. That was the dinner-table conversation in my house.

B: What? That your parents were talking about different issues?

P: Yes. My mom, for example, became CNO when I was about 20. I was still in college and she was a director at [another institution] for a long time before that. She actually changed things; she's one of the people who started the Critical Care Consortium in Seattle. She was a pretty big person in this area, though not so much now. For example, she was one of the first people at [her institution] to start wearing street clothes as a supervisor. [Before she came along,] you had to be a director, so that was a big thing. She was willing to change things, and she's the one that thinks like that. My dad does, too, but my mom more so. Now she's at a private hospital, so it's very different from this hospital. Her ideas were always helpful to me because they are totally different from what anybody would say here.

B: And it gives you a different perspective?

P: Yes. She would say, "You need to fire that person." I would tell her, "I can't do that, but I can do this. . . ."

B: It's that element of creativity, which is, in a sense, openness to new ideas.

P: I think "constraint free" is a really nice way of saying it. When I first started, I was in here with my first RN3 and she and I are totally different. We took the Myers-Briggs [personality inventory.] We were totally different on every single thing. She was more of the overachiever—just read every journal and just lots of good things about her. She was just a little bit more rigid than me, and she would always say that she couldn't even fathom the ideas that I would bring up. So it was fun to play off of that [aspect] of each other, but it made me realize, "Oh, my ideas are kind of weird sometimes."

B: It sounds like your parents were not so much mentors, but certainly models in the field. Have you had a mentor in this system, in this setting?

P: When I was an RN3. What ended up happening was that we had an acting nurse manager. She's from Five Southeast, and we are Five Northeast, and we see the same patients. They are ICU and we're not. She's a nurse manager over there and I was acting [nurse manager] over here; she said, "I'll help you." I didn't really want to be the acting nurse manager. I was pretty happy being an assistant nurse manager, so I was kind of "pep talked" into it. I was pretty content. I didn't realize that I would like it better. That had not happened yet. [Other managers said,] "We'll support you." I really relied on [the other nurse manager] heavily and talked to her every day: "What about this, blah, blah, blah." And she was so nice to me, just letting me talk and [being supportive:] "That sounds fine; try it out." Because there really is no answer to anything—you realize that especially as time goes by. She was very patient with me, and I really, really appreciated that. I got the job and then shortly after that, she became my boss. She's still my boss, which is so lucky. She knows my unit; she knows my style; she helps teach me her stuff. It couldn't be any better for me.

B: She actually had been consistent during the whole time since you were acting nurse manager?

P: And I can still talk to her.

B: If you can sum up some things that you took away from that relationship that you translated in your own way to your work as a nurse leader, what would you say?

P: The number one thing is that people need support when they're in a big change. Just that availability of someone to talk to was huge for me, so I [try to] provide that to other people. In terms of actual operational stuff, though, do you mean?

B: Leadership, how she dealt with people, problem solving—those kinds of things. What did you see in her that you have crafted and taken on as your own?

P: [. . .] Some of the stuff—for instance, the budget—I just see it as kind of a concept. I'm not a numbers-oriented person. [My boss] encouraged me to try things. She was into the IHI [Institute for Healthcare Improvement] initiatives where you would just try something, just do it. It's health care proven. For example, for a quality plan, she said, "Just do it in two rooms and see if you like it. Then, if you do, you can branch it out bigger." You get over your fear of starting something.

B: She was really attracted to change, comfortable with it, as well as the idea that you just sort of jump in.

P: And [she taught me] how to make [change] manageable, which was huge. It's incredibly helpful. She was learning it, actually, while she was teaching that to me. It was so great.

B: [She advocated] the model that, when dealing with fear, it is best just to go ahead and jump off and see what happens.

P: The worst thing you could do [was wait.] We all made fun of our academic setting. You could spend two years literally [waiting]. I could think of five examples of this—of trying to get something for free and put it out there. And that's just what we don't want to do: wait two years to start this thing. So get a team together, involve the nurses, and then go for it. Try something, just try it. Everybody knows once you try it, then you realize, "Oh, we're not done with this; we're done with this." It's a whole different thing. All your issues become different, and then you are actually moving forward.

B: So [your role models were] this person in this setting who started with you as an acting director and then also the example of your parents as you were growing up.

P: I could always call if I was really puzzled about anything. And you know my dad, just as much: He's the one who really gave me a pep talk to go and fight for this job, because I thought I couldn't do it. He said, "Of course you can do it." You know, he always thinks that I'm the smartest person ever. I truly have wonderful parents. He's great at doing the pep talk. I had a lot of mentors along the way. And my husband supported me, too.

B: I want to talk about one particular experience, what we call a high-point experience—a sort of a standout moment, just one time where you just felt alive and engaged in the flow, as they say. You didn't want to be anyplace else. What did that look like, sound like, and feel like?

P: [. . .] We had one RN3 who was very high performing but a little bit scary. She was scary because she was working so hard—maybe two shifts of overtime a week. Just remember that this was a really bad staffing time. When people would do something that wasn't that great, she would just be so frustrated with them. People respected her because she worked so hard and yet felt like "Watch out!" It was things like "You mean you didn't read that board I put up? What am I doing here, if you guys aren't even going to read the board?" She was very brutal. That was my biggest stress when I first started, just that working relationship, even though we had been friends. Her stress level was so high. I had to tell her, "You can't do any more overtime. You're getting too grouchy." This is somebody who oriented me and was the person who hired me back.

So here is my high-point moment: She left. The whole time she and I were working, I had another RN3 position [open]; it was my old position. I couldn't fill it because nobody wanted to work with [the RN3 who departed]. That was obvious, and I'm not sure that she ever figured it out. As soon as she left, I had two full FTEs of RN3s. I can't remember who had the idea—somebody had it, but I don't think it was me—of posting three part-time positions instead of two full-time positions. I still have two FTEs of RN3s, but I filled them with three people because they all work part-time. I think it was because the people I really like work part-time and I wanted to attract them desperately. But I also think somebody else thought of it because I thought, "Oh my God, that's a great idea." I could remember that—just realizing the potential there.

We have the ability to transform this unit. We're at the beginning of a new time. I remember thinking that when the original person was giving me so much grief: "I am going to outlast you. I'm going to be here when you're not here, and we're going to see what this unit is like then." It was very stressful; I don't want to go into that.

I posted the positions and got the interview teams together, interviewed people, and hired them. I really felt like I need to rise; I need these people with whom I've worked since I was a new graduate to see me as a manager in this role—not to just come in here thinking I'm taking over the office. I need to actually say, "I'm going to be a leader and I'm going to help you guys." It was a little bit of "we're going to frame what it's going to look like for the future." Now I see us working flat, but I also didn't want to go into that to mamby-pamby.

B: You wanted to be really clear about what the boundaries were.

P: Right. I wanted to show my leadership capabilities at that point. You know, it's like you can just feel the opportunity, and I wanted to rise to it. I put a lot of thought into how I did every step of it. We hired three people to start on the same day. That was really a big change; it was a huge change. But it was a really positive change. I wanted to take that and run with it. Even if I just went forward and didn't change anything, it would have been an improvement. But I really didn't want to just go flat; I wanted to go like that—and we totally did.

We have a consultant in our organization in the training area, and I asked him to come and do retreats with me and the new RN3s. I had heard that one of my peers had used the consultant to work with her management team when they were having problems. She was having some conflict and struggles within their management team. I thought, "I should do that at the beginning so that we're all on the same page, and so that we don't end up having conflicts later." I really didn't worry about that, but I like the idea of having this conversation when you really figure out what you want in the future and what is possible and that kind of stuff.

The awkward part was that the person who left wasn't really gone: She was giving notice, and she was going to overlap for three months. I think that was stressful for them, but it was also important because she needed to hand off some pretty big stuff to them. That was probably the most awkward part about it. You could see her thinking, "Oh my God, times are changing."

B: She could see it transform before her eyes.

P: That's right, and then she could see herself phasing right out. It was positive that she had something else going, and was going to be fine. That was really interesting.

We had retreats. We talked about why we go into nursing and what inspires us and so on. What do you see for the unit? We had already recovered some from our lowest point, but we weren't where we are now—not by a long shot. We were still hiring a lot of people. We hadn't done much about team building yet with the staff. You know when you're in survival mode, you can't team build when your team's not the same from one week to the next. I put a lot of work into making sure [the new nurses] had good orientation. I made sure each of them got what they needed, and we would meet once a week. I wanted to make sure they reached their goals. I was in total heaven, trying to teach them all the things I think are fun. They all have their own strengths because we're all different in here, which is great.

B: When you think about the high-point aspect, part of [it] is that joy of a novel solution, and taking advantage of the potential of the situation and being able to see a future that would be really different—that had a lot of potential. What else personally engaged you at that time?

P: I loved mentoring those guys.

B: Bringing them along and teaching them what they needed to learn?

P: Each one of them at their first evaluation was in tears. Each one of them.

B: Because they . . . .

P: They said, "This is harder than I thought it was going to be, and I want to do this and I'm only this." It made me nervous because I wanted them to be happy, but to each one of them I basically said, "That's just how it is. You know, we're going to do a little bit, and then maybe it helps a little bit. Then you do something [else], it does help a lot. Then you do something else, and it helps a lot. That's just how this job is. And you have to accept that. You're not going to get all the CNAs to be perfect within six months. It's just not going to ever happen. But we'll always get a little bit better, a little bit better, a little bit better." I think I helped them. I mean you don't want to squash anybody's spirit.

B: No. You want to acknowledge their frustrations, while at the same time you verbalize your resilient overall framework.

P: I probably even said to them, "This is why you're in this job. You can see the gloryland of what it would be if it was perfect." You don't ever want to lose that.

B: Right. It's like a vision of what you're striving for along the way.

P: That's right. And it's not a reflection on you as a person if we don't go right there. I mean, they really take it personally because they are high-performing people. I was trying to depersonalize it a little bit and say, "What makes you good or not is whether or not you keep trying. Try something different; don't do the same thing over and over again if it didn't work. [But maybe] five years later, you pull it out and it works then."

B: So the key is being able to teach them some of the things and model for them some of things you identified as your strengths—resilience and big-picture thinking. Something that came up before [in other interviews is having a non-judgmental nature and not taking things] personally. You haven't really talked about that for you. Is that an element of your strength?

P: I think that is a way to not put yourself through the stress mill. And I think it's appropriate.

B: If someone told you, "You don't take this personally, and I really do; this stuff really gets to me," what would you say to them?

P: Usually, if you can take apart the situation and even just use work language, you can help get rid of that feeling. One of my RN3s got blasted by a night-shift nurse one time. It was devastating to her; she ended up going to counseling later. There's nothing I can do to make that go away. It just drove me crazy. I just thought, "This is a reflection on her and where she's at in her work. If she's attacking you personally, it's still about her. You still need to go back to 'I'm in this role; I'm doing the best I can.' Her needs aren't met for some reason, and we can figure out what's wrong with them, but it's not about you. Maybe you should get feedback on how you are performing, and that's fine." I say in work language, "She has a performance issue,"—just to use some of those words—and "We're going to help her with that. She's having problems communicating her feelings without becoming personal or whatever." I just think in some ways if you can rephrase it, you can see it for what it is. It's like work; it's a professional situation.

B: The vocabulary that you use somehow introduces a little bit of distance where it's not so personal.

P: If you operated on that level all the time, you just wouldn't be able to function at all. What she was learning from that [experience]—she talked about it recently—was that "I can try as hard as I can and people still won't think I'm doing great all the time." And that's something for management people to get used to. It's true because you get criticized "just because." We had one nurse here who was very anti-management. It got to the point that you could have a perfectly good relationship with her, but if she was going to have a choice, that was the way she was going to go. It could be the way she was raised or [something else], but [the negative attitude] was there. You do figure out it's not about you. You still have to listen for feedback. People are wishing I was out there talking to patients more. I hear that. I'm fine with getting feedback.

B: It's being able to pull out the piece that really is about you and that you can learn from and then trying to take it in a nonpersonal way. You were talking earlier about how you teach people how to do that. How does it work for you? You just gave a little tidbit.

P: That was my big learning over the first [months in the nurse manager role], and that's probably my parents helping me through that, because they've had so many experiences. When I first started—you know, people love to be very critical. I was so new and I had done things "wrong." You get into conversations where people are just taking you apart. I learned how to respond to that. I can switch it and say, "We're not talking about me" or "You told me that. Now you've given me that feedback, is there anything else that you would like to tell me right now? Because otherwise this conversation is over. I'm not listening to this for half an hour."

B: So some of it was setting a boundary about it, and some of it was listening to the part that's actually true?

P: If I can get the person talking to me to say, "So you wish I would do this . . . ." Yes, "I wish you'd do this," instead of listening to 20 minutes of "You're such a disappointment to me." I don't get that now, but I did back then. I just learned how to stick up for myself.

B: You would say that?

P: Yes. I remember one person I accidentally forgot to cross off who was sick. [That person was listed as] a no-show, and it was totally my fault. The nurse said to me, "This just shows how you don't care about the unit; you don't even realize the impact." I said, "Don't talk to me like that. I am working 40 hours a week for this unit because I care about it. I made a mistake, and you can tell me that. That was a really awful day, and I hear that. I'm sorry. I'll do everything I can not to do that again, but do not talk to me like I don't care about the unit. I don't appreciate it." And she sent [her criticism] to me as an e-mail. I told her not to e-mail me stuff like that. If you want to talk to me, you can talk to me—but this, to me, is not professional.

B: So it's also a form of self-assertion to what you have to say.

P: Yes. I wasn't born like that. I'm pretty much going to be more like, "Oh, it must be my fault." I probably will tend toward that [self-effacement.] I had to grow that part of me that says, "Hey, wait a minute! I'm doing the best I can here. You can give me feedback and I'll hear it, but don't act like I'm not trying." That's what I didn't like.

B: It is that balance between listening for what's real and then drawing the line between what's abusive or not true about you—and you're not going to stand for that. You do that yourself and model it. Now I want to go back to your staff nurses. Describe a time when your partnership with a nurse made a difference in the care of a patient, where you helped a nurse with patient care. What factors were present, and what was your contribution? Just describing a time of a partnership with a staff nurse.

P: It happens all the time on a small scope. I think my biggest thing is going to be that you don't judge the patient—just try to think of what they need. What I'm drawn to thinking about is the times when the patient had a complaint and I was drawn into [the situation].

I can think of one example. It wasn't one particular nurse, though. It was more like the team. We had a patient who was very dissatisfied with his care from the medical team. Things we were doing weren't really helping, but the main need that wasn't being met was not being met by his physicians. How do you work with that, because you don't want to say, "Well, it's not us." This patient's needs weren't being met, and his wife was just in tears. He didn't seem to be thriving. He had a surgery, and it's two weeks later and nobody comes to see him anymore. I spent a lot of time with his wife. We pulled together a care conference where the nurse was there and came up with things. This is where creativity comes in: "What will make this better for you?" I think I'm role modeling to the nurse the different things you could think of. I think that's something I'm pretty good at, because I really do want the patient to feel better. "You know, if you just stick with that . . . ." I don't try to make excuses or argue with a patient.

This patient needed to see his doctor more often, so there were things that we negotiated with the service. We actually got a different service. That made all the difference in the world. He went home three weeks later. It was just a great moment. [Part of the family's complaint was] "People are talking so loud in here. We're a very quiet family. We don't talk loud like that." We put up a sign saying,

"Please talk quietly when you enter the room." It was probably things like that: What would make you feel more comfortable? People needed to know the plan when they came in the room so that they didn't make it worse.

B: Everybody knew the plan. So in collaboration with that nurse, [you figured out what the family wanted and helped] to implement that.

P: That continuity part is a little hard for us, but you just put paper all over the place. You know, "Here's the plan." We showed it to the family and the patient: "If we did this stuff, would it help?" [We said to staff members,] "We're going to put this in the Kardex and you guys are all going to talk to people. Then just try to make sure that everybody is approaching [this plan] when this patient is not getting his needs met." That's a lot different than "This patient and family are a pain; they are needy." I always think it's interesting when thinking about the concept that they've lost trust in us. When somebody's lost trust in us, everything's important. We have to go overboard. We will do anything we can think of, because if this was your grandpa and he was actually scared to be here, what would you want? [The patient and family] need to see that visible change and us acknowledging that their needs weren't met. And [the patient's] poor wife was just terrified that he was going to die—and he didn't, he lived. Part of his component was anxiety, so a change in the doctors was probably the biggest change, but then we were part of the supporting role in meeting his needs.

B: In relation to a different topic, your interface with senior leadership is obviously important to your role. Can you give me an example when an administrator or senior manager helped you succeed? It would be at another level than what you just described. Can you think of a time like that?

P: So many times. If I think of [name deleted], I can remember her bringing up something that she wanted us to do and us being able to say, "Seriously, don't make us do that." The nice thing about this hospital is that the managers have a really good sense of consensus: We have the same values. We like primary nursing, and we like giving education to the nurses. There's things that you could ask any of us, and we would all immediately agree on. That's a nice place to work.

[In this case, we all said], "You don't know what this is going to do to us." And [in response, she said,] "I'm listening to you, and we're not doing it. We might have to do it differently, and we'll think about that." Moments like that.

Here is an example, even though it wasn't so much [the supervisor]. It had to do with the work hours that nurses worked. There was going to be a change because of the new union contract, and [the supervisor] really stepped up and talked to the nurses. She had open forums all the time. She listened to them and helped work out a negotiation with the union that met their needs.

B: The overall theme, then, is responsiveness to your needs and listening.

P: Listen and believe me.

B: So there are two questions along this line. Can you recall a time when you felt support by your organization?

P: Here's probably the biggest turning point. My director is [name deleted]; she's the one who was my [original] mentor and still is. We were in this horrible staffing situation over the past couple years. It was just horrible, and it was not getting better. Well, it was getting better really slowly. I can't remember what was going on—maybe we didn't want to use travelers because of the budget or something. Anyway, [my director] made it so that the timing worked out so we could close beds. Nobody thought that we closed beds for staffing, but rather that when we closed those beds, it was because of low census or something. We closed beds and that saved us. It totally saved us. If we had to be open, we had to staff our floor—and we would fill up and then we'd go back down. Even with a low census, we'd fill up and then go back down to 22 [beds], go back up to 30 [beds], and go back down to 22 [beds]—and that's just exhausting. But we also didn't have enough nurses for that. So [the director] decided to strategically close 4 beds. I can't even remember what the actual supposed reason was. I think it was because of low census: "We're going to have to do this for low census and close beds all over the hospital." That [decision] was crucial because at that moment our staffing got better. I mean, just the minute you closed those beds, our staffing was appropriate—more appropriate for the amount of nurses we had. We were able to slowly reopen, but only when we got enough people.

There's junctures like that where you think, "I don't think I can do this job anymore." I am not going to manage a unit [where we have only] 19 FTEs when it needs to be 40. I am not going back to that.

B: So [your example is the director] intervening because she sensed the impossibility of [the situation] and finding a way to do it?

P: This hospital does not close beds for staffing [reasons]. We would not have then, and I don't think we would do it now. It's not in our culture—but she found another way to do it.

B: Her message to you was, "I understand you're overwhelmed here and I will do everything that I can."

P: She has, at the right moment, been there for me. Staffing was horrible, and I think it might have been my first Joint Commission survey as a manager. I got called and told that night shift was short and I needed to come in. I came in at 3:00 a.m. to take care of patients, and that was the day Joint Commission was coming. I was ready to cry. You can just imagine how much work I had done the week prior. I was totally exhausted, and I really hated the feeling of being at the whim of my work. Not against anyone else, but I could not say, "No, this was my job." They would not have called me at that point if there was another idea. We had been through all that stuff. I came in thinking, "This job sucks and I can't believe I'm doing this." The Joint Commission [survey] went great. I got in here, and I found a coffee cup with candy in it and a note from [my boss] stating, "Thank God for you." It was perfect timing. I was ready to . . . I was thinking, "This is not worth it and I am just getting abused." It really made a difference to me.

B: Let's extend this to the bigger picture. How has this particular organization been a good fit in enhancing your success here and your longevity?

P: I appreciate the focus on Magnet [status], the academic setting, and the importance given to the research. For example, we wanted new thermometers. IC studied a pair and determined which thermometers were working best. They weren't happy with the literature. They found two and picked one, and they supported that purchase. We got all new thermometers for the whole hospital. We really didn't have money for that, but we were doing it. Ours is sitting in here somewhere; they haven't been put up yet. And I fought for this—I really did. These are the moments where I really do make a difference, [but they] really won't be remembered by anybody but me.

B: But you have the satisfaction of knowing your impact?

P: That happened when we were sitting in those meetings talking about those thermometers. I was part of that group for two years. I said, "We can't just have nine. We need one in every patient's room." The reason was because they wanted us to wipe them off every time, and I felt like that was totally ridiculous. It sounds so small for someone who is not a nurse. What's the big the deal? You have to stop and put gloves on, and you have to get the wipes, and you have to wipe [the thermometer] off, and then you have to throw [the wipes] away, and then you have to throw your gloves away, and then you have to wash your hands. Nobody is going to do that every time they go in and out of a room; it's just never going to happen. So I'm not implementing something that's never going to happen [even though] we know we have it in [writing as a] practice. You [say something] like, "Well, I hope people do this, but I don't want to put in a new [procedure] with full knowledge that nobody's going to do it." Everybody [realized,] "That's ridiculous. Think how much money that is." I was just fully holding firm to that. Of course, I talked my other medical/surgical nurse managers into agreeing with me. Pretty soon, everybody was saying, "We need one in every room." It was a lot more money; it was like three times more money.

I was telling my mom about it after, and she said, "That's an interesting battle to pick." I said, "Yes, but I just don't want to put [into the hospital procedures] one more thing that people don't do." She didn't feel it was that big of a deal, but I thought it was.

We did it. I don't think anybody would go back and say that it was me who thought of that, and I don't know for sure that I am the only one who thought of it. But I sure thought it was important, and we are getting it, and the nurses are going to love it.

B: When we started with the question, "How is this organization a good fit?," one of your answers to that was responsiveness, the other was decisions made based on research.

P: Right, evidence-based research. [My hospital leaders] are putting their money where their mouth is. We talk about research all the time. It would be very easy to say, "Oh, that's not so much research that you [need to put computers] in every room." It was more the process of picking it and agreeing to buy [the technology].

B: But [your leaders] are backing you up. Anything else about this place that is a good fit for you and has contributed to you being here?

P: I have really appreciated the flexibility of being able to change my schedule around. I don't think nurse managers can do that everywhere.

B: In your case, what you do mean by "changing it around?"

P: For me, I work four "tens" [10-hour shifts per week] during the summer, so I can spend more time with my kids. They are 9 and 11 years old. That's actually a pretty big deal to me because I have worked full-time ever since they've been born. I've been at this job basically that whole time, and I appreciate the flexibility. If I needed to get to an assembly at two o'clock, I can do that. I couldn't do that if I was on the floor. It's nice.

B: It's highly unusual in this role.

P: I wouldn't even think that it wouldn't be that unusual, but here's the [most important] part: I thought, "I'm totally missing out on my children's childhood." Both of my sisters are stay-at-home moms. I was really worried that I would regret what I was doing—you know, somehow I would regret it, right when I was at the crux of that. I think my youngest was three or something. I felt like, "He's going to start school." . . . I was just not sure I should do this or not. I was really torn and didn't really like my job and was in the middle of a really cool project. I was working a lot.

I never work more than 40 hours a week, by the way. I know nobody says that, but that's true for me. Most nurse managers, either they work 50 or 60 hours or that's what they always say. But I'm always honest about the fact that's not me. I told [my supervisor], "You can hire me, but I'm not working more than

50-hour weeks, just so you'll know." If there was something going on that needed it, I would do it. I don't think that comes around that often.

Somebody had started talking about working four tens [4 days of 10-hour shifts per week], and that totally swung the thing for me. And here are two things: One, I started taking off Tuesdays so I could hang out with my pre-schooler before he started school. I had a good eight months before he started school where it was just he and I one day a week. That was weird for him, because he was used to always being with his brother. It just really, really meant a lot to me. I didn't get that with my older son, but that's okay because it all came around when it needed to.

[Second,] I thought, "What does a stay-at-home mom have that I don't have?"—and that was that they are standing at the door when the kids come out of school. So then I started working 7:00 to 3:30 or 6:30 to 3:00, and I would be there. I did that for a whole school year, I think. I would actually be there and stand there and pick them up. I don't think I did it every single day, but I think I did it two days out of the week and then two days I would work 9:00 to 5:00. I don't like to get up early, anyway, so I was not going to push it that hard. And then I'd be able to be here for later meetings and stuff, so I'd switch which days they were going to be. Just the fact that I could do that two days a week [meant] I didn't feel like I was missing out from what the rest of the mothers were doing.

B: So it's a form of support from this organization: Flexibility is a way of communicating, "We know that the rest of your life is important, too," and there may be times where you can switch it around for that. And you have.

P: Knowing that I would still do my work, and I would and I did.

B: Well, that's communicating and [showing] faith in you.

P: It really doesn't matter to me. I mean, I don't feel like it really matters what your hours are: It's getting the work done. A lot of times, some of those innovative hours are more efficient. I personally feel like four tens are probably the most efficient hours for a manager because you get here a little earlier. It forces me to get here earlier. So you see days, evenings, and nights [shifts] for a little chunk of time, and you get a little more work done because you get done with whatever the normal meetings would be and you're going to have two more hours.

B: That's interesting—it ends up being more efficient.

P: But this hospital is talking about getting rid of it [the current scheduling system] right as we're speaking, so I'm irritated right now. But it has been something, and my boss wants to give it to us. It's something coming from somewhere else. I'm going to get to do it this summer, and I don't know what's going to happen next year. It may make a huge difference to do that summer stuff—to go hang out at the pool all day. I'll take off a week at Christmas so my kids don't have to get out of their pajamas on the day after Christmas.

B: Just a quick one: Do you think that [flexible schedules] contribute to your being able to renew yourself when you do that?

P: Yes, I definitely do. I wouldn't tolerate it if I didn't feel like it was; I did tolerate it for a while.

B: You'd feel too torn?

P: Yeah, I think I would have quit, I really do—because there is nothing more important to me than my kids. I would have had to figure out something else. So, yes, it does make me feel more renewed.

B: Two more questions, and these are both speculative. If you could have three wishes for new nurse middle managers coming into the field, what are your three wishes for them?

P: I didn't talk about it, but I also got to go to every class that they have—team building, communication, conflict resolution. I went to everything.

B: So your wish is?

P: That they [new nurse managers] would be able to do that. Have the adequate education, feel supported in going to education things. Not start off too busy. One [wish] would be education; [another wish] would be to make sure that they have a reasonable situation they are walking into. If they need staffing, make sure that they have the staffing. Support that. In my scenario, I feel like I was supported: Even though we were in a bad situation, I had that support to work on it and to do what we needed to do. I was supported to do the things I needed to do until we got our own staff.

B: So they [the hospital leaders] had the foresight to see you coming and know what you needed to make that a better way.

P: No, I had to figure it out. I had to figure it out, but I got support when I asked for it. No, I learned the hard way how to make sure the unit was covered.

B: Okay—so education, getting people the backup that they need, and what else?

P: Giving them enough money in their budget to be able to do different things. You need to have a little bit of leeway to try different things.

B: If you had four wishes?

P: I was just going to say that I think people should be able to start off slow a little bit.

B: Let the pace pick up over time.

P: If they are new, they should have a mentor, somebody who's right there. If you need something, you go to them and you can talk to them. Somebody just came up to me and said this; I need to talk to them this afternoon. This person will have time to talk to me.

B: Is it a designated mentor? It's not someone who you hope you'll find.

P: It's a designated mentor. They would never hope to find [a mentor] in that state. I can't imagine somebody finding a mentor on their own. And the other thing is, I think the rest of the managers should be the [fall-back] mentors to a new person. So, if there is one main person, but so and so is really good at explaining the budget, and so and so is really good at figuring out conflict and personnel issues and this and that, everybody should have an open-door policy. And I did experience that.

B: Do you tell the nurse managers that? Do you tell them who to go to for their needs?

P: Yes, absolutely. They should stay tight with that person. I heard later—years later, after I hadn't been new—"Oh, I wish I would've had that support." Well, I just assumed I had it. I walked up to ask people stuff, and I got the help I needed. I think partly it comes from the person, but I also remember saying, "[Name deleted] is really good with the budget. Go meet with her for two hours and she'll explain it to you."

B: So if you could build that in—if not everyone is an initiator the way that you are in looking for the support they need to make in this connection—designating a mentor and letting people know?

P: You can just designate [your interest by saying,] "I'm really interested in this and I'm happy to talk to people about it." Then let them say what they like to talk about. Put that out there for people.

B: That's sounds good. Now your last question: Driving home from work today, you slip through a wrinkle in time and it's the year 2015. At this time, all the vacancies for nurse managers are filled, average tenure is ten years, and nurse manager satisfaction is the highest it's ever been. What would have happened to create this change?

P: [The main consideration] is if the patients and the nurses are happy, then the managers are going to be happy. So it's letting the nurses and patients have what they need and letting the manager be the one—not necessarily the only one—who is effective in getting those things to the nurses or to the patients. And I think the same, if you asked me what would make for better nurse satisfaction: Make the patients happy. That makes the nurses happy, and that makes the nurse managers happy.

Number two, I think their salaries should be decent. If you can be effective with nurses and the patients, and make a decent amount of money, and have flexibility in your work schedule—those are my top three. But I think there are other things—professional practices—[that are important to] the nurses being happy. I really care about that. I love working in an academic setting. . . . I just feel so lucky. That part makes you feel proud to work here. It's things like that that make you feel you are working in a special place.

B: Those were all my official questions. Is there anything else that you wanted to add on this whole issue of your own engagement and vitality as a nurse? Is there anything that you wanted to mention that we haven't covered? We've really covered a lot of ground, and you're a wonderful storyteller. You're very reflective about what your strengths are, which makes it really great for me because I can really see with clarity. I can imagine you out there doing what you do and, more importantly, what some of your habits of mind are as you are doing it. Anything else you want to add?

P: I think it really is a great job. I think about the fact that I am getting my master's degree and I am almost done. I think I want to stay in this job. I like it.

B: It's the right fit for you.

P: Yes. You know, you can get too far away from the nurses and you're not having as much fun. I don't even know what happens to people when they go to different areas. Like somebody who comes in from QI; you see them, and they look kind of miserable. I don't know why that happens. Someday I'll find that out.

Index

A

Accessibility of information and resources, 58–59

Accountability
  of nurse managers, 76–77
  of physicians, 76–77

Achievement in success of staff, 27–28

Adams, John, 37

Administrative support, availability of, 68–69

Affirmative framework, 10–11, 45–48, 50
  curriculum for, 89

Ambiguity, coping with, 44

American Organization of Nurse
  Executives (AONE), 2

Applications of NMEP findings, 6

Appreciative inquiry methodology, 4–5, 73

Ardor, 8–9, 24–27, 50

Assumptions, setting aside, 42–43

Attunement, 10–11, 40–43, 51
  curriculum for, 89

Autonomy
  of nurse managers, 61
  of staff, 23–24

B

Balance, work–life, 78

Bedside care. *See also* Patient care
  and management behavior, link between, 17

Behavior modeling, 47–48

Bennis, Warren, 18

Big-picture thinking, 18, 20

Boundaries, emotional
  internal, 33
  modeling and displaying, 32–33
  restoring, 34–35

Boundary clarity, 8–9, 32–35
  curriculum for, 89

Bowcutt, Marilyn, 45

Bracketing, 42–43

Brand pride, 70–71

Burn, David, 89

Burnout, avoiding, 78

Business assistants, 79

C

Calling to nursing, 24

Change
  emotional mastery of, 11
  seeking, 44–45
  welcoming, 44

Change agents, 12–13

Change agility, 10–11, 43–45, 50
  curriculum for, 89

Chief nursing officers (CNOs), signature
  behavior evaluations, 49–54

Child care on campus, 78

Clinical instructors, 79

Colleagueship, 76–77